MEDICAL KNOWLEDGE
Doubt and Certainty

prepared by the U205 Course Team

THE OPEN UNIVERSITY
Health and Disease   U205   Book II
A Second Level Course

THE OPEN UNIVERSITY PRESS

The U205 Course Team

U205 is a course whose writing and production has been the joint effort of many hands, a 'core course team', and colleagues who have written on specific aspects of the course but have not been involved throughout; together with editors, designers, and the BBC team.

Core Course Team

The following people have written or commented extensively on the whole course, been involved in all phases of its production and accept collective responsibility for its overall academic and teaching content.

Steven Rose (neurobiologist; course team chair; academic editor; Book VI coordinator)
Nick Black (community physician; Book IV coordinator)
Basiro Davey (immunologist; course manager; Book V coordinator)
Alastair Gray (health economist; Book III coordinator)
Kevin McConway (statistician; Book I coordinator)
Jennie Popay (social policy analyst; Book VIII coordinator)
Jacqueline Stewart (managing editor)
Phil Strong (medical sociologist; academic editor; Book II coordinator)

Other authors

The following authors have contributed to the overall development of the course and have taken responsibility for writing specific sections of it.

Lynda Birke (ethologist; author, Book V)
Eric Bowers (parasitologist; staff tutor)
David Boswell (sociologist; author, Book II; Book VII coordinator)
Eva Chapman (psychotherapist; author, Book V)
Andrew Learmonth (geographer; course team chair 1983; author, Book III)
Rosemary Lennard (medical practitioner; author, Books IV and V)
Jim Moore (historian of science; author, Book II)
Sean Murphy (neurobiologist; author, Book VI)
Rob Ransom (developmental biologist; author, Book IV)
George Watts (historian; author, Book II)

The following people have assisted with particular aspects or parts of the course.

Sylvia Bentley (course secretary)
Steve Best (illustrator)
Sheila Constantinou (BBC production assistant)
Ann Hall (indexer)

Rachel Hardman (designer)
Mark Kesby (illustrator)
Liz Lane (editor)
Vic Lockwood (BBC producer)
Laurie Melton (librarian)
Sue Walker (editor)
Peter Wright (editor)

External Assessors

Course Assessor

Alwyn Smith President, Faculty of Community Medicine of the Royal Colleges of Physicians; Professor of Epidemiology and Social Oncology, University of Manchester.

Book II Assessor

Charles Webster Director of the Wellcome Unit for the History of Medicine, University of Oxford.

Acknowledgements

The course team wishes to thank the following for their advice and contributions:

Sheila Adam (community physician) North West Thames Regional Health Authority.
John Ashton (community physician) Department of Community Health, University of Liverpool.
Herman Berrios (medical historian) Robinson College, University of Cambridge.
Ralph Colp, Jr. (psychiatrist and historian) Columbia University, USA.
Kate Hunt (human scientist) Department of Community Medicine and General Practice, University of Oxford.
Ludi Jordanova (historian) Department of History, University of Essex.
Klim McPherson (medical statistician) Department of Community Medicine and General Practice, University of Oxford.
Anne Murcott (sociologist) Department of Sociology, University of Cardiff; Department of Psychological Medicine, Welsh National School of Medicine.
Margaret Pelling (medical historian) Wellcome Unit for the History of Medicine, University of Oxford.
Hilary Rose (sociologist) Department of Applied Social Studies, University of Bradford.
Janet Sayers (psychologist) Department of Sociology, University of Kent.
Simon Schaffer (historian of science) Department of History and Philosophy of Science, University of Cambridge.

The Open University Press, Walton Hall, Milton Keynes MK7 6AA.

First published 1985. Copyright © 1985 The Open University.

Designed by the Graphic Design Group of the Open University.

Typeset and Printed by the Pindar Group of Companies, Scarborough, North Yorkshire.

ISBN 0 335 15051 9

This text forms part of an Open University course. The complete list of books in the course is printed on the back cover.

For general availability of supporting material referred to in this book please write to: Open University Educational Enterprises Limited, 12 Cofferidge Close, Stony Stratford, Milton Keynes, MK11 1BY, Great Britain.

Further information on Open University courses may be obtained from the Admissions Office, The Open University, P.O. Box 48, Walton Hall,

About this book

A note for the general reader

Medical Knowledge: Doubt and Certainty is the second of a series of books on the subject of health and disease. The book is designed so that it can be read on its own, like any other textbook, or studied as part of U205 *Health and Disease*, a second level course for Open University students. As well as the eight textbooks and a Course Reader, *Health and Disease: A Reader**, the course consists of eleven TV programmes and five audiocassettes plus various supplementary materials.

Open University students will receive an *Introduction and Guide* to the course, which sets out a study plan for the year's work. This is supplemented where appropriate in the text by more detailed directions for OU students; these study comments at the beginning of chapters are boxed for ease of reference. Also, in the text you will find instructions to refer to the Course Reader. It is quite possible to follow the argument without reading the articles referred to, although your understanding will be enriched if you do so. Major learning objectives are listed at the end of each chapter along with questions that allow students to assess how well they are achieving those objectives. The index includes key words (in bold type) which can be looked up easily as an aid to revision as the course proceeds. There is also a further reading list for those who wish to pursue certain aspects of study beyond the limits of this book.

* Black, Nick *et al.* (eds) (1984) *Health and Disease: A Reader*, Open University Press.

A guide for OU students

Chapters 1–3 of Book I, *Studying Health and Disease*, introduced the basic methods used in biomedical science. Book II, *Medical Knowledge: Doubt and Certainty*, develops this and introduces two new themes. First, adequate medical knowledge requires the social as well as the natural sciences — a fully biosocial approach. The second theme concerns the broader nature and consequences of scientific advance in medicine. What are its origins? How far has it transformed our beliefs? Has it had costs as well as benefits?

These two themes are illustrated through four case studies. The first (Chapters 2 and 3) contrasts modern approaches to health and disease with those of traditional cultures. The second (Chapters 4–6) considers an infectious disease, plague, and its changing relationship to human society. The third (Chapter 7) surveys contemporary debates over a mode of treatment, hysterectomy. And the fourth (Chapters 8 and 9) reviews historical and contemporary attempts to understand a mental condition, hysteria.

When you have completed the book, you should return to Book I, *Studying Health and Disease*. A biosocial approach to health and disease entails a grasp of social as well as natural science methods.

The time allowed for studying Book II is three weeks or 30 hours. The table overleaf gives a more detailed breakdown — to help you to pace your study. You need not follow it slavishly but do not allow yourself to fall behind. If you find a section of the work difficult, do what you can at this stage, and then rework the material at the end of your study of this book.

Study time for Book II (total 30 hours)

Chapter	Time/ hours	Course Reader	Time/ hours	TV and audiocassettes	Time/ hours
1	$\frac{3}{4}$				
2	4 $\Big\}7\frac{1}{4}$	Loudon (1984)	$\frac{3}{4}$	TV programme: *Images of Health* $\Bigg\}$	$1\frac{1}{2}$
3	$3\frac{1}{4}$	Dubos (1979)	$\frac{3}{4}$		
		Helman (1978, 1981)	$\frac{3}{4}$	Audio sequence:	
		Illich (1976)	$\frac{3}{4}$	*Images of Health*	
4	$\frac{1}{2}$ $\Big\}5\frac{1}{4}$				
5	$2\frac{3}{4}$				
6	2				
7	3				
8	$2\frac{3}{4}$ $\Big\}4\frac{3}{4}$	Smith-Rosenberg (1972)	1		
9	2				
10	$\frac{1}{2}$				

Assessment There is a TMA (tutor-marked assignment) associated with this book; three hours have been allowed for its completion.

Contents

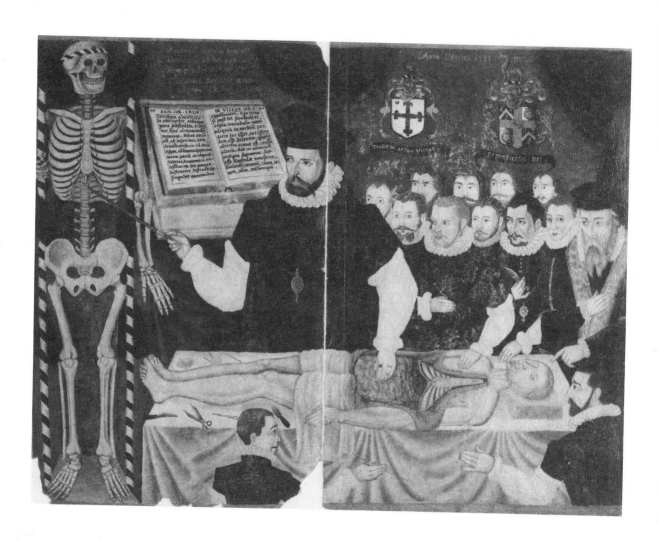

An anatomy lesson in 1581 at the Barber-Surgeon's Hall, London.

1
Introduction

When a problem presents itself 'not accountable for but upon Hypothesis, we should restrain our Judgement, and leave the doubt to be solved by Posterity, when they shall have obtained Light enough from Experiments which have escaped us. It therefore behooves us to defer our Opinion about the uses of the Spleen ... the Causes of Contagious Diseases from Poisons, etc, till Time shall bring the Truth to Light. By this means Physic, tis true, will be reduced to a small Compass but then it will be true, certain and always the same.' (Boerhaave, 1708, quoted in Shryock, 1979, p.68)

This ringing vision of science and the scientific method in medicine (or Physic) was written by the great Dutch physician, teacher and chemist, Herman Boerhaave (1668–1738), who worked at the University of Leyden. At the time that Boerhaave wrote, there was little that medicine could do for most diseases. A patient with diabetes could sometimes be diagnosed, but nothing was known of the cause of the condition, nor were there any successful treatments. Much the same was true of almost every other disease; even the diagnosis was usually uncertain.

How did we get from there to where we are today? What are the steps by which humanity was able, if not to conquer disease, at least to begin to understand its many forms and to mitigate some, though not all, of the worst of its effects?

   ☐ Part of the answer is contained in the quotation from Boerhaave. What does he suggest?
   ■ That, if we want to make serious progress, we should concentrate on small, manageable, cautious steps. There is no need to try to solve everything at one go. Some tasks can safely be left to those who will follow us. We ourselves should stick with what we can be certain of.

This vision of the scientific method is, therefore, based on an essentially *sceptical* or *empirical* attitude towards human knowledge. On this view, many of the things that we think we know are merely beliefs, not *knowledge*; they are not things whose truth is certain. To be certain of that truth we need to test it, and that testing is a slow, painstaking, and often painful process. But the pains are worth taking; for certain knowledge of the way the world works, knowledge of which we can be sure, is a powerful thing. It is the only certain way to limit the much greater pain that disease itself can cause.

It took a long time to obtain practical facts in medicine, and it took even longer for people to be convinced that there was anything in this cautious approach to topics like death and disease. People desperately wanted answers right away; they did not always want people like Boerhaave saying not to worry, that posterity would find out in the end. Nevertheless, the cautious approach did eventually catch on. Boerhaave did not find out very much, but some of his successors did. This book tells the story of the rise and eventual triumph of scientific medicine. The sceptical but practical approach was pursued in many countries but came of age in France in the nineteenth century. It was there, in Paris, following the Revolution and the Napoleonic reforms, that modern medicine was firmly established for the first time. No previous doctors had been as sceptical as the French; no previous doctors were as successful. The guidelines laid down by the French and their German successors had, by the end of the nineteenth century, set a pattern for medical science and medical practice which is still with us today. With the success of the new science, doctors' prestige rose to heights that had never previously been achieved in the long history of medical practice. Two hundred years after he wrote, Boerhaave's vision had come true.

The creation of medical science is a heroic story, one of which all human beings can be proud. It is also something from which we can still learn. That is why it is so often told. That is one of the reasons why we shall tell it here. And yet, as with most good stories, there are several alternative versions — versions which also must be told. Boerhaave thought that there would be *progress* in medical science only if scientists were duly cautious in the way they theorised about the body and its workings. A similar caution can prove equally fruitful in our more general reflections upon health and disease. It may pay us to be sceptical about at least some of the ways we think about modern medicine and some of the claims that are made on its behalf. We should also cast a wary eye on some of medicine's critics, too. We shall focus primarily on just one form of medical science, the science that has been developed by clinicians and natural scientists, biomedical science or *biomedicine*.

This book has two main themes. The first is the development of medical science, the lessons we can learn from it, the progress that has been made and the various doubts about some aspects of that progress. The second is the fact that medical science has both a biological and a social nature, and only by taking a fully *biosocial* approach can we hope to reach a proper understanding of the issues that confront us. These two themes are both illustrated by each of four case studies. Consider our first topic: the contrast between modern and traditional medicine. Chapter 2 focuses on one half of medical science, the biomedical side, and traces its rise from the Greeks to the present day. In doing so, it illustrates the theme of human and scientific progress. But Chapter 3 then introduces another and perhaps equally important approach — that of *socio-medicine*, and in particular *anthropology*, the comparative study of cultures. Doing so raises a few queries about the extent of our progress — have we come quite as far as we sometimes like to think we have? Perhaps some of our faith in biomedicine resembles the magical beliefs of previous eras?

The next case study takes a slightly different tack, and tries to show how biomedical explanations are more plausible in this instance than socio-medical explanations. Plague was once the scourge of humankind. The Black Death in the fourteenth century is estimated to have killed between a third and a half of Europe's population, and it was to return again and again until the eighteenth century. What caused its arrival and eventual disappearance? Traditionally, most historians have felt the answers lay in social and economic change. More recent analyses, however, suggest that the answers lie first in biological mutation and second in the development and application of biomedical science.

The case studies on hysterectomy and hysteria present a rather different perspective on epidemics, and in doing so allow the introduction of some further aspects of the critique of modern medicine. Bubonic plague was an epidemic, a sudden spread of disease in a community. But an epidemic need not necessarily be caused by microorganisms. George Bernard Shaw, an acute observer of the medical profession, once remarked that fashions were merely epidemics induced by tradesmen, but that 'the psychology of fashion becomes a pathology' when epidemics are produced by doctors.

Can doctors actually produce epidemics? There are two related answers to this question. First, medical treatments may themselves have harmful effects. Treatments can, therefore, constitute a form of disease and, if they become fashionable and spread rapidly throughout a community, they too can be classified as epidemics. Is the huge rise in the rate of hysterectomy a *surgical epidemic*? This question is considered in Chapter 7. Second, some of the 'diseases' which doctors treat turn out not to exist or to be of extremely contentious status. What counts as a disease at one time may be denied at another. In consequence, just as there can be epidemics caused by viruses, and epidemics of fashionable treatments, so there can be *diagnostic epidemics*, great waves of supposed 'disease' which sweep across the community as new crazes take hold in the medical trade and in the population at large. Hysteria, the topic of Chapters 8 and 9, is now claimed by some to be such a disease.

What causes these fashions, if such they are? Hemlines go up and down, lapels get narrow or broad, hula-hoops come, skate-boards go. All of us seem prone to crazes of one kind or another. But these seem trivial compared with health and disease, and the critics of medicine have discerned some dark motives. Shaw, writing of the medical fashions of his day, thought that money was the answer. This is still a powerful argument: the financial reasons for the extraordinary differences in the number of hysterectomies performed in Britain and the United States are considered in Chapter 7. More recent critics of medicine assert that there is a yet more dubious cause; for them, medicine provides a means of *social control*, a method by which the power of some is reinforced at the expense of others.

Women have made particularly forceful criticisms of both contemporary and traditional medical practice. To some feminist critics, medicine is merely an agency of male control and oppression: for them, hysterectomy consists of men cutting out women's wombs, and hysteria is either a condition produced by women's subordinate status, or else merely a figment of male doctors' imaginations, a repressive device to further men's power over women. How far these arguments are true will be examined in some detail. As you will see, even the counter-arguments make rather more pessimistic assumptions about the nature of medical knowledge than are held in the triumphalist account of scientific medicine.

Finally, a note on this book's title — *Medical Knowledge: Doubt and Certainty*. 'Doubt and Certainty' reflects the two opposing themes — on the one hand, the slow but powerful growth of scientific knowledge, on the other, the many doubts that still surround both our knowledge of health and disease and some of the uses to which medicine can be put. 'Medical Knowledge' requires more extensive comment. The word *medical* is often taken to refer exclusively to doctors. Medical knowledge is thus the sort of knowledge that doctors possess, or think they possess. But there is an important sense in which everyone has medical knowledge to a greater or lesser degree, for everyone is a doctor at times:

> Between friends, I think every man of tolerable parts ought at my time of day, to be both doctor and lawyer, as far as his own constitution and property are concerned. For my own part, I have had an hospital these fourteen years within myself and studied my own case with the most painful attention. (Matthew Bramble in *Humphrey Clinker* by Smollet, 1967, p.52; first published 1771)

Matthew Bramble, Smollet's hero, is a 55-year-old 'valetudinarian', a splendid, old-fashioned word for someone who worries a bit too much about their health. He spends his time touring round fashionable spas in search of a cure for his gout. Yet his words apply to everyone, at any age and whatever their condition. All of us are ill on occasion and examine our condition with great attention just as, to rephrase Smollet, everyone has a hospital within them. Moreover, just as we sometimes study our own case and minister to our own condition, so we are often obliged to care for the health of others, women particularly so in our society. Most illness is minor and most of the doctoring that is done is not done by doctors; they are called in only when the illness gets more serious. Even then, we are still expected to do a fair bit ourselves. In other words, those formally designated as doctors are merely the professional end of the spectrum of medical care. Their learning is certainly specialised but it overlaps with, influences, and is in turn moulded by, the wider medical practice of which it is a part. The study and the critique of medical knowledge concerns the knowledge that each and every one of us possesses.

2

A new science; a new faith

Towards the end of this chapter you will need to refer to the Course Reader for the article 'The history of pernicious anaemia from 1822 to the present day', written by Irvine Loudon (Part 1, Section 1.6).

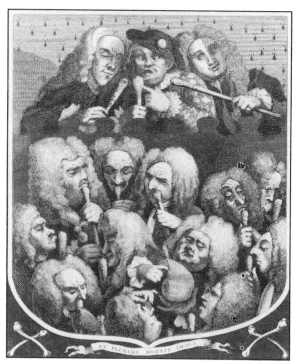

Figure 2.1 'A Consultation of Physicians' by William Hogarth (1736).

Let us continue tracing the rise of biomedical science by going back a hundred years or so before Boerhaave's sceptical but ultimately hopeful approach to medical knowledge, this time not to a doctor but to a shrewd observer of the medical profession, the French philosopher and essayist, Michel de Montaigne (1533–92). Montaigne too was a sceptic, but of a more pessimistic, sixteenth-century kind. The new philosophy, of which he was a part, called all in doubt; traditional knowledge was held in great suspicion. Montaigne, however, was sceptical about the future as well as the past, for he had a firm grasp of the *complexity* of both the natural and the social world. He therefore had little faith in the possibility of serious medical knowledge; of medical science as we would now call it. Let us see what he has to say about the medicine of his time and the problems it found:

> For the rest, I honour doctors, not, as the saying has it, out of necessity . . . but for love of themselves, having known many decent and lovable men among them. My quarrel is not with them but with their art, and I do not greatly blame them for making their profit of our stupidity, for most people do so . . . .
> . . . [The doctor] is faced with so many maladies and so many circumstances that before he has attained certainty about the point that the successful completion of his experiment should reach, human wit is wasting its ingenuity. And for him to find among that infinite number of things, that the right cure is this elk-horn; among this infinite number of diseases, epilepsy; among so many constitutions, the melancholic; so many seasons, in winter; so many nations, the French; so many times of life, old age; so many celestial mutations, at the conjunction of Venus and Saturn; so many parts of the body, the finger . . . he would have to be guided by a perfectly regular and methodical fortune. And then, even if the cure seems to work, how can he be sure that this was not because

the illness had reached its term, or a result of chance, or the effect of something else he had eaten or drunk or touched that day, or the merit of his grandmother's prayers? Moreover, even if this proof had been perfect, how many times was the experiment repeated? How many times was that long string of chances and coincidences strung again for a rule to be derived from it? (Montaigne, 1580, pp.305–7)

☐ What is Montaigne's main reason for being so sceptical of medical knowledge?

■ His central point is that the world is too complex for doctors to possess either an accurate diagnosis or any serious proof of the efficacy of their cures.

☐ If this is so, why then do many people still have faith in doctors, according to Montaigne?

■ They 'honour doctors ... out of necessity', that is, because they are sick and have no alternative.

To trust doctors, or healers of any kind, is difficult, for it is to grant them a special power over our lives. The newly diagnosed diabetic, for example, may be expected to engage in meticulous assessment of everything they eat and of the exercise they take; a complete change of diet; regular medical examination; and, perhaps, daily injections and routine monitoring of the sugar level in the blood or urine. This is power indeed, power that stems from *authority*. The nineteenth-century German historian, Theodor Mommsen, called authority of any kind 'more than advice and less than a command, an advice which one may not safely ignore'. It can be hard to ignore medical advice, not usually because of any physical or legal threat by the healer but because of the consequences that the healer predicts will ensue if the advice is rejected.

How the practice of medicine came to be associated with science, the development of effective medical applications of that science and the effects on medical authority are the subjects of this chapter. However, first it is worth considering in some detail just how recent is the rise of medical science, how different the situation of doctors used to be, and how, in consequence, they were forced to rely on a good many other methods of reinforcing their authority. Some of these traditional methods still remain, as you will see, for science by itself is not sufficient. Nevertheless, the change that science created in doctors' overall position has been so dramatic that it is now hard to imagine the much lower status that many doctors held, even in the nineteenth century. Here, for example, is a passage from the historian Theodore Zeldin, which describes the position of French doctors and *healers* in the mid-nineteenth century, precisely the time and the place where medical science was first established on a firm footing. Yet, as Zeldin shows, the authority of the average doctor was very far from secure:

The visitor to Paris in 1848 would have found some 1,550 doctors there, 300 of them decorated with the Legion of Honour, offering every variety of cure. At least 50 per cent of them would have published books to advocate their theories and many of them advertised in every available medium. Dr. Bachoni offered electro-physico-chemical treatments with no payments if no result. Dr. Barras offered a modification of the Broussais doctrine, replacing gastritis with gastralgia as the cause of all ills. Dr. Becquerel offered cures for stammering in conflict with those of Dr. Jourdan, with whom he conducted public disputes. Dr. Belliol's name covered the walls of Paris and the small advertisement columns in the papers offering "a new vegetal method". Dr. Leuret, author of *The Moral Treatment of Madness* (1840), though refuted by Dr. Blanche and voted against by the Academy of Medicine, persisted in tying his mad patients to planks of wood and throwing cold water over them ....

Dr. Jean Giraudeau of Saint Gervais did not just cover the walls of Paris with his name, but paid newspapers to praise him and hacks to write books for him .... Phrenology (and also physiognomy and cranioscopy) ... had academicians and professors teaching it, and applying it to education, jurisprudence and medicine .... The "microscopists", "pharmaco-chemists" and "numerists" (applying statistics to the study of disease) met with vigorous opposition ... and the medical press attacked and ridiculed every idea, new and old, and every personality in the same slanderous and uninhibited way as the political papers. In the country, doctors had to fight the even more powerful resistance of superstition and traditional remedies. A whole army of rival practitioners offered cheaper and sometimes more acceptable treatment: the urine healer (who prescribed medicines after examining the urine of the patient), the orviétan merchant (the itinerant seller of drugs), the sorcerers, the nuns, the priests, the old women, the midwives, the pharmacists .... In 1911 a doctor describing popular medicine in the Vendée reported that the doctrines of Broussais still had many fervent followers. Bone-setters still made a good living and died well-to-do, bequeathing their secrets to a chosen disciple on their deathbed. Magical and herbal cures, distributed by clairvoyantes, were much used; special trains were organized to take large crowds to holy places, where every disease was cured by miracles. Babies were given wine or eau-de-vie to make them strong. Madmen were considered to be the victims of curses and the Devil ....

... The position of the doctors was ambivalent ....

Only to a very limited extent was it a way of rising in the world, partly because those who entered it needed a lot of capital to obtain the education, and partly because it seldom yielded high rewards. Charton's *Guide to Careers* of 1842 stressed the heavy expenses involved and the poor rewards, 'Some can obtain an honest living but most will obtain a mediocrity of position which is really hardly encouraging.' [see *Punch* cartoon, Figure 2.2] .... To succeed in the upper ranks of the profession (Charton noted) needed more than brains: 'nepotism, favouritism, camaraderie are carried to the highest degree'.
(Zeldin, 1973, pp.25–31)

☐ Comparing this picture with that of modern medicine, what can you tell from it about: (a) nineteenth-century French doctors' status and that of their rivals; (b) the prestige of science in the nineteenth century; and (c) doctors' relationships with one another?

■ (a) Most doctors seem to have been much poorer on average than they are today, to have had far less social prestige and to have faced a good deal more competition from rival sorts of healer.

(b) The passage reveals how, though all these doctors disagreed with one another, they all still claimed to be 'scientific'. Everyone wanted to wear the mantle of science and benefit from its authority. Note also that some scientific aspects of medicine are still recognisable, if often by another name, such as the 'numerists' (or statisticians), but that other doctrines have disappeared or been absorbed, for example, phrenology (a form of psychology based on the analysis of the brain and skull). The content of science changes over the years.

(c) Finally, you may have been struck by the ferocity of medical competition. Modern doctors do not advertise, nor is the medical press full of ridicule and personal slander.

One of the most striking things about the passage from Zeldin is the extraordinary diversity of the medical systems on offer. Nowadays, most doctors claim authority by virtue of their training in an agreed body of knowledge, a common curriculum of recognised theories and facts, taught in legally recognised institutions. How far there is, in fact, agreement over that knowledge may be questioned. It certainly changes over time. There may well be a major difference between, say, old general practitioners trained at an ancient teaching hospital and the recent generation produced at a new, more community-oriented medical school. Moreover, there are still doctors today who take up an interest in hypnosis, homeopathy and acupuncture; three fashions which were also evident in Paris in 1850.

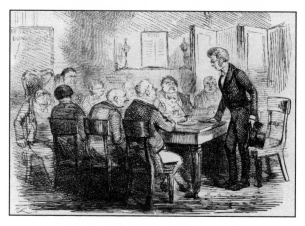

Figure 2.2 Splendid opening for a young medical man.
CHAIRMAN   Well, young man. So you wish to be engaged as Parish Doctor?
DOCTOR   Yes, gentlemen, I am desirous —
CHAIRMAN   Ah! Exactly. Well — it's understood that your wages — salary I should say — is to be twenty pounds per annum; and you find your own tea and sugar — medicines I mean — and, in fact, make yourself generally useful. If you do your duty, and conduct yourself properly, why — ah — you — ah —
(PUNCH   Will probably be bowled out of your situation by some humbug, who will fill it for less money.) (*Punch*, 1848)

Nonetheless, although there is still variety, modern medical expertise has an essentially *collective* nature; the doctor's authority mainly derives from being specially trained in a body of knowledge which is stamped, supposedly, with the seal of science.

This is knowledge to be trusted, or so it is claimed; the best that hundreds of years of research can produce. The actual content of the knowledge changes, of course, over the years, as yet more is discovered about health and disease. No doctor is completely up to date in every area and no doctor claims to be. There is instead an extraordinarily elaborate division of labour. Some doctors — the general practitioners — are generalists, whereas others specialise and do so in an extraordinarily minute way. Yet each can keep in contact with all other doctors, and with the knowledge they possess, through weekly journals of research and comment, through magazines which specialise in updating, through meetings and conferences and training programmes, and finally through referral. A doctor who is uncertain about what exactly ails a patient has an enormous variety of colleagues who can provide a second opinion; and if the colleagues themselves are not certain, the patient may be passed on to yet more specialist centres.

The idea of a body of trained professionals sharing collectively in the best scientific knowledge of their day and drawing their medical authority from their membership of this group or 'college' took root in Italy in the late fifteenth century. It was at first restricted to a tiny, academically trained élite of healers but, as university medical education broadened in Europe and America, from the mid-nineteenth century onwards, the proportion of healers specifically trained in this body of knowledge increased dramatically. Over time, therefore, more and more medical practitioners were embraced by the professional, scientific ethos and recognised as members by the accrediting bodies, which guarded access to the college, patrolled what was to count as knowledge, and expelled those found guilty of unprofessional conduct. At the time of which Zeldin mainly writes, the 1850s, the Academy of Medicine was clearly an important authority in France, but it was not the only one, and it was itself riven by many violent personal disputes. Many of the doctors whom Zeldin mentions claimed to follow their own *personal* system; each offered a unique way to better health. Instead of the dominance of *academic medicine* and the relatively uniform product which it offers, there were innumerable systems from which patients could choose if they had the money.

Something of this variety still survives today in private medicine. Financial competiton between doctors produces an appeal to a more personal authority than is normally found within a State-run system such as the British National Health Service. But this more individualised style is a pale shadow of its former self. Private practitioners may still be rivals but their competition is severely restrained by the ethos and standards of biomedical science on whose wider authority every practitioner must draw.

The replacement of the personal competitive form of medical practice by the more collective style of medicine today owes something, perhaps a great deal, to the gradual extension of the academically trained doctors' *legal monopoly* of certain kinds of practice; a process that began in Renaissance Europe and was dramatically broadened in the nineteenth century. In an important way, modern medical authority derives from membership of a tightly controlled trade union or guild, a 'closed shop'. Indeed, critics of professional medicine have long argued that its authority is merely a confidence trick, a restraint of trade, a legal manoeuvre, a conspiracy between medicine and the State. All these arguments bear some examination but they do not completely explain just how the trick was pulled off. Even in the United States, whose traditions were fiercely opposed to such legal monopoly, professional medicine eventually got its way. A powerful argument can be made that the ever-widening scope of professional medicine, the legal certification of its particular brand of knowledge owes something, perhaps a very great deal, to the dramatic advances in the scientific understanding of health and disease that were made from the Renaissance onwards. Not only were many old mysteries solved, but their solutions often made, as we shall see, a striking impact on public opinion. Disease has always been feared. Those who have means to cure or prevent it can usually claim a major reward. However, though at the time of Zeldin's account many doctors certainly claimed the mantle of science, the authority of the Academy, such authority was relatively weak compared with that of present-day medicine.

☐ Re-read Zeldin's description and list the other main sources of authority on which French healers tried to draw.

■ French doctors appealed to the verdict of the public via open debate; to their personal authority; to favourable book reviews; and to the medium of advertising, a new method of getting their names known. More traditional healers appealed to more traditional forms of authority: to religion; to craft skills, such as bone-setting; to traditional herbal remedies; to old-established systems of medicine, such as urine analysis; to folklore; to magic; and to the experience of age.

☐ Can you think of any other means of generating authority which healers might also use? What other things can impress people when they visit a doctor?

■ There are three other major sources of authority which often do the trick. First, there is a distinctive personal style — a good 'bedside manner'. Second, there is the healer's wider social status. In a hierarchical society, for example, a healer from an élite background may carry some of the general authority of that élite. Third, people may be impressed by distinctive apparatus, unusual clothes, mysterious bottles and instruments.

Take the issue of bedside manner. Consider the following pieces of professional advice offered by various medieval doctors:

Dress soberly like a clerk, not like a minstrel. Keep your finger-nails well shaped and clean.

Do not walk hastily, which betokens levity, or too slowly, which is a sign of faint-heartedness.

Tell the patient that, with God's help, you hope to cure him, but inform the relatives the case is grave. Then, if he dies you will have safeguarded yourself. If he recovers, it will be a testimony to your skill and wisdom. When asked how long recovery will take, specify double the expected period. A quicker recovery will redound to your credit, whereas if a patient finds the cure taking longer than prophesied, he will lose faith in your skill. If he asks why the cure was so swift, tell him he was stronghearted and had good healing flesh; he will then be proud and delighted.

(quoted in Turner, 1958, p.15–6)

Medical students are still instructed to dress soberly like clerks and warned of the professional dangers both of levity and of telling the patient precisely what they think. So some means of generating authority have stayed much the same. Moreover, since Western doctors are drawn largely from middle-class backgrounds, this too may lend them an air of authority over many of their patients. In the past too, social status was drawn upon heavily, though sometimes in a rather different way. The outsider might generate even more authority than the member of the élite. Rasputin, the favoured healer at the Court of Nicholas, the last Tsar of Russia, never washed or changed his clothes and had the style of an outcast and mystic. Likewise, in the late eighteenth century, the American Indians had a major reputation as healers in the United States; so much so, that some of their white competitors tried to pass themselves off as 'Indian doctors'.

More conventional doctors, however, took, or tried to take, the high rather than the low road to healing power. There were still some heights to which they could not aspire. The best example of the medical virtues of high status is the traditional British cure for the 'King's Evil', or 'scrofula', a form of tuberculosis. The ideal cure was to be touched by the monarch; see Figure 2.3. Dr Johnson, the eighteenth-century literary critic and compiler of the great English dictionary, used to recall being taken as a child all the way from Lichfield in Staffordshire to London for this treatment. Ordinary doctors could hardly be King. They could, however, attempt to be gentlemen. Aspiring eighteenth-century English physicians dressed fashionably and carried a gold-topped cane. A doctor's riches might indicate that, surely, he had something special to offer. A character in the eighteenth-century magazine, The Spectator, remarks of a poor doctor: 'Go send the knave about his business. Was his business as infallible as he pretends he would long before now have been in his coach-and-six.'

To sum up: in an age before medical science was particularly effective, and when relatively few healers belonged to the academically trained élite, most doctors relied heavily on other modes of generating authority. They often claimed to be scientific but they might also stress, where they could, their wealth, their status, their culture and their manners. Many advertised their expertise with vigour and savagely disputed the claims of their rivals, both inside and outside the profession. Doctoring was fiercely competitive, often disrespectable and always vulnerable. Much of this was to change radically. Not all the old tricks of the trade have entirely disappeared but those that remain are less important than they used to be. Most doctors now claim to share in a collective body of scientifically generated knowledge. How a major part of that knowledge was created, the biomedical part, is the subject of the next sections. Even Montaigne might be partly persuaded.

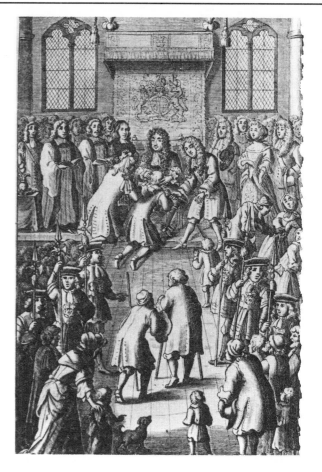

Figure 2.3 Charles II touching sufferers from scrofula (The King's Evil).

Science versus speculation

How did this new science come about, the science based on close observation and careful experimentation, the cautious, painstaking but ultimately optimistic approach that Boerhaave had praised? There are different ways of approaching this question. Some place its origins in the major religious upheavals that shook Europe in the sixteenth and seventeenth centuries, in particular the rise of Protestantism; others see both scientific and religious change as symptomatic of a more fundamental political and economic transformation that was gathering speed at this point, the birth of modern capitalism itself.

These ultimate causes are not our concern here. We shall focus instead on some of the intellectual changes that occurred within science itself and on a few of the key people who played a part in the creation of modern biomedical science. This way of telling the story, the focus on 'heroes' and 'heroines' and the 'breakthroughs' that they made, has some important drawbacks — difficulties that will be considered at the end of this chapter. But it is also much the easiest way to introduce you to the subject.

So, bearing this caveat in mind, let us begin with the classical tradition. Modern Western science has many important precursors among the classical civilisations of the Greeks, the Chinese, the Arabs and the ancient Egyptians. European medicine has, for example, traditionally hailed a Greek doctor, Hippocrates of Cos (*c*.450–*c*.370 BC) as its founder. Cos is an island opposite the ancient city of Cnidus in mainland Turkey. In the fifth and fourth centuries BC both these places had famous medical schools. Their doctors engaged in close *observation* and investigation of disease and treatment, published detailed case histories and made extensive critical comments on one another's work. How far any of Hippocrates' own work survives is not known, for most of the work of these two schools is anonymous. However, a very considerable body of their writings still exists and has exerted an enormous influence over the practice of Western medicine; indeed, the main theories which they espoused were not to be finally overthrown until the nineteenth century.

Even though there is very little in this work with which modern medical science would now agree, Hippocrates and his colleagues may reasonably be classified as scientists, for they believed in close empirical study of health and disease and reasoned argument. This was at least a beginning. However, some modern critics of ancient science have described it as a series of brilliant taxi-ing runs in which the aircraft never actually took off. The empirical work of the Greeks was certainly added to over the centuries, first under the Roman Empire, particularly by the Greek doctor and anatomist, Galen (AD *c*.129–*c*.200), and then by various Arab doctors such as Ibn Sina (Avicenna) (*c*.980–*c*.1037) and Ibn Rushd (Averroes) (*c*.1126–*c*.1198). However, the scientific tradition never became self-sustaining. Only a few undertook new investigations and, over the centuries, most scholars merely codified their predecessors' work, which came to be treated as gospel rather than as a mixture of more or less interesting observation and speculation. Academic doctors looked back to the great texts of the past. Unlike Boerhaave, they had no vision of themselves or of later generations actually adding to this body of knowledge. In other words, there was no conception of scientific progress.

Much of this medieval reverence was justified. The medical tradition which had reached most European universities by the fourteenth century from the Arab writers was far in advance of anything then extant in Europe itself. But the reverence was taken a good deal too far. Francis Bacon (1561–1626), the leading Renaissance philosopher of science, wrote thus of medieval scientists:

. . . who having sharp and strong wits, and abundance of leisure and small variety of reading, but their wits being shut up in the cells of a few authors (chiefly Aristotle their dictator) as their persons were shut up in the cells of monasteries and colleges and knowing little history, either of nature or time, did out of a great quantity of matter and infinite agitation of wit spin out unto us those laborious webs of learning which are extant in their books. (Bacon, *The Advancement of Learning*, 1605, quoted in Quinton, 1980, pp.25–6)

☐ What, according to Bacon, should scientists stop doing? What should they do instead?
■ They should stop purely abstract theorising and get out of their colleges and monasteries and into the world.

Bacon's enemy was empty *speculation*. Purely armchair study could not, by itself, lead to serious knowledge about the world. Scientists had to look for themselves. There were also other aspects to this new vision of science. Paracelsus (1493–1541), a Swiss medical practitioner and chemist, had urged alchemists to turn from their dreams of making gold and look instead to the making of new medicines. Bacon put his more general vision of science in the following terms:

Of myself I say nothing; but on behalf of the business [Science] which is in hand, I entreat men to believe that it is not an opinion to be held but a work to be done; and to be well assured that I am labouring to lay the foundation, not of a sect or a doctrine, but of human utility and power. Next I ask them to deal fairly by their own interests . . . join in consultation for the common good . . . come forward themselves to take part in what remains to be done. Moreover, to be of good hope, not to imagine that this Instauration [plan of the sciences] of mine is a thing infinite and beyond the power of man, when it is in fact the true end and termination of infinite error. (Bacon, *The Great Instauration*, 1620, quoted in Quinton, 1980, p.18)

☐ How does this differ from (a) the view of Montaigne about the possibility of scientific knowledge, and (b) the picture of the relationships among French doctors in the nineteenth century cited earlier?
■ (a) Montaigne was sceptical about the possibility of any systematic medical knowledge; Bacon was merely sceptical about traditional beliefs.

(b) In Zeldin's portrait, the French doctors were selling their own personal medical systems. In Bacon's vision, however, science is a fundamentally cooperative collective enterprise, one in which each scholar contributes to a common whole.

Some of the Greeks too had seen science as useful, had emphasised detailed observation and mutual criticism and learning. What made Renaissance science different was the way this approach penetrated to the very heart of some societies. Galileo was persecuted by the Catholic church but Francis Bacon was the leading lawyer of his day and Lord Chancellor of England, as well as a philosopher of science. When a new scientific society was founded in London in the seventeenth century, it was under Royal sponsorship and had Charles II as a member. Nonetheless, for all this prestigious sponsorship, it took a long time before the scientific point of view was firmly established within medicine. To make a beginning in physics was relatively easy compared with the intricacies of biology. Disease was a highly complex matter, as Montaigne had pointed out. Effective medical science had to wait until the nineteenth century. Spectacular advances in anatomy and physiology, such as Harvey's discovery of the circulation of the blood (1628), were certainly made early on, but these were hard to apply to medical problems. As a result, medieval (ultimately classical) theories predominated until the nineteenth century. Scientific advances still occurred within medicine but they were largely incorporated within the framework inherited from the Greeks.

The essence of the classical tradition was very simple. There was held to be just one cause of all morbid phenomena, one pathological condition which explained all disease. Bacon had talked of medieval scholars who 'out of no great quantity of matter spun their laborious webs of learning' and this was an accurate description of most medical theorising until the nineteenth century. Physicians took a few facts and on this simple basis created ingenious and enormously complex theoretical systems in which they tried simultaneously to explain all forms of sickness and to show that *every* form had just one underlying cause and required the same basic treatment. A theoretical system which ascribes everything to one ultimate cause is an example of *monism* (though this term has other meanings as well). Medical monism came in two main forms: one, known as *humoral theory*, ascribed all sickness to an imbalance of bodily fluids; the other, known as solidism, to an imbalance of forces in the solid parts of the body resulting in tension. F.J.U. Broussais (1772–1838), the French doctor mentioned in the quotation from Zeldin, argued that everything was due to gastroenteritis, and C.F.S. Hahnemann (1755–1843), the German founder of homeopathy (the last of the major monistic systems), reduced nearly all pathology to the 'psora' or itch.

These monistic theories of cause were accompanied by equally simplistic theories of treatment. Systems which revolved around theories of fluid imbalance treated disease by trying to remove the unsatisfactory fluids through bleeding, purging (using powerful laxatives), blistering, vomiting and sweating. Those which, on the contrary, saw sickness as the result of tension in the more solid parts of the body used somewhat different methods. John Brown (1735–88), an Edinburgh doctor whose system proved extraordinarily popular throughout most of Europe and the Americas, had merely two treatments: large quantities of whisky as a stimulant or, when relaxation was held to be necessary, large quantities of opium.

By the eighteenth century, monistic theories of bodily tension were of some importance. Albrecht von Haller (1708–77), the Swiss teacher and physiologist, had conducted major research into the working of muscles and this had led to a shift towards theories based on the solid tissues of the body. But throughout most of the preceding period, academically trained doctors had favoured theories of the bodily fluids, or *humours* as they used to be known. Indeed, we still speak of people as being 'in a good humour'. Humoral theories probably stemmed from European folklore but were developed by the Graeco-Arabic medical tradition. The names of the four humours survive in English as descriptions of temperament or character: melancholic (yellow bile), phlegmatic (phlegm), choleric (black bile) and sanguine (blood). These humours were linked in a complex theory to the four 'elements' — earth, air, fire and water — and also to the related four 'qualities' — wet, dry, hot and cold. People's behaviour was seen as due to a difference in the mixture of these elements and qualities, and whether or not they were in balance. The human body, like everything in the cosmic order, was thought ideally to exist in equilibrium but when this was disturbed, sickness manifested itself, for example, in the erupting boils of the choleric. Traditional medical treatments sought to restore the balance.

Put another way, the classical medical view of health and disease was primarily *holistic*. It was the era of what was then termed the *sickman* — in other words, medicine was focused on the whole human being. Illness was seen as a total psychosomatic disturbance, involving all aspects of both the mind (psyche) and the body (soma); everything was out of balance. As such, it was the classic era of bedside medicine; the doctor visiting patients in their home, talking to them and studying them in a highly individualised fashion.

Let us now briefly review the major changes that have occurred since then, before going on to describe them in more detail. By the nineteenth century, with the advent of the new science that Bacon and Boerhaave had foreseen, the sickman had begun to disappear (Jewson, 1976). The patient was now a case rather than a person. Illness was no longer regarded as a total disturbance of mind and body, but as a highly specific *disease* consisting of an abnormality in the tissues of a particular organ. The characteristic setting of advanced medical practice shifted from the patient's own bed to the hospital ward where cases were gathered together in large numbers. It was only then that doctors began to think in *statistical* terms; not of the unique characteristics of individual patients, but of the frequency of this or that condition. Finally, whereas the traditional doctor tried to estimate the future course of the sickness — its prognosis — and apply a cure, the key medical task of this era was the diagnosis and classification of illness. Sceptical of all forms of therapy, doctors merely concentrated on the systematic description of disease.

The period from the late nineteenth century to the present day has seen both a continuation of the progressive localisation of disease within the body and a partial return to the more holistic model of the sickman. On the one hand, therapy has come back into fashion and specific cures are now sometimes available. Moreover, the site of advance has shifted from the hospital ward to the laboratory. The prime concern is no longer with organs or tissues but with biochemistry; the patient is no longer a case but a cell-complex. But, on the other hand, the body is now also seen in *homeostatic* terms, as a self-regulating system which maintains an internal balance in various essential processes. Moreover, there is a growing awareness of the psychosomatic, of both the social context and the inseparability of mind and body. Medicine is thus uneasily poised between extreme *reductionism** and a return to holism, though a holism of a rather different kind from that of the classical and medieval tradition.

This quick sketch of the main changes in medical thought is a very primitive guide to what actually happened. Real life, as the quotation from Zeldin illustrates, was a good deal more complex than that. Nevertheless, it should provide something to steer by as we begin to explore the impact of science upon medicine.

The classification of disease
Some aspects of the medical approach to disease are explained in *Studying Health and Disease* — in particular, how the attempt to construct a stable classification of different diseases ultimately fails.

☐   Why is this?
■   Because, as medicine learns more and more about different diseases, so it continually modifies their classification.

* Reductionism is the approach to understanding through breaking things down into their constituent parts. Holism, as its name implies, argues that things can be understood only when viewed as a whole. These concepts are discussed more fully in *Studying Health and Disease*. The Open University (1985) *Studying Health and Disease*, The Open University Press. (U205 *Health and Disease*, Book I).

There is, therefore, a sense in which 'diseases' are purely human creations liable to change as human knowledge changes. However, important though this lesson is, there is another sense — some may think it more important — in which diseases have their own reality, quite independent of the way anyone thinks about them. Whether or not our classification is correct, they can kill us all the same. Much of the success of scientific medicine has been based on the way it has been increasingly able to specify the precise nature of different diseases; to grasp each in ever more detailed empirical form. No system of disease classification is ever going to be perfect, but some systems are a lot better than others. The scheme first developed by clinical scientists in the seventeenth century was a huge improvement over the traditional form of classification and it has been systematically improved ever since. So great an improvement was this scheme, and so revolutionary in its implications, that it is hard to grasp the old way of viewing disease.

☐   What was said earlier about the difference between the traditional and the modern ways of thinking about disease?
■   In traditional medicine, there was only one disease; in scientific medicine, there are many.

This achievement, like the others discussed in this section, was the work of many people but is typically associated with the name of Thomas Sydenham (1624–89). Sydenham was virtually self-educated as a physician. He had not undergone the standard academic training of his day. This very lack of training, coupled with his receptivity to the ideas of sceptical authors such as Bacon may well have led him to a new approach to disease, though one shaped also by earlier doctors such as the Dutch physician, J.B. van Helmont (1579–1644):

> Where the classical physician wrote of disease, Sydenham wrote of diseases. Where the ancients had seen an inseparable connection between the patient and his malady, Sydenham saw in the patient certain pathological symptoms which he had observed in others and expected to see again. In a word, he distinguished between the sick man and the illness, and objectified the latter as a thing in itself. (Shryock, 1979, p.14)

Sydenham left excellent descriptions of measles, dysentery, syphilis and gout, all written in a plain, matter-of-fact style — itself a novelty. Here was a really significant advance. John Locke, the seventeenth-century philosopher who was also a doctor, saw great promise in the method. 'I wonder', he observed, 'that, after the pattern Dr. Sydenham has set them of a better way, men should return to the romance way of physic.' Unfortunately, the 'romance' or speculative way was to continue for some time. For, though careful clinical description worked well with a few clear-cut conditions, the description of other diseases proved far more controversial. Not only were enormous numbers of 'diseases' identified (Francois de Sauvages (1706–67) described 2 400), but there was no general agreement on the classificatory systems. Moreover, by itself the method did not present a decisive challenge to the traditional monistic theories. The traditionalists could still argue that this great variety merely reflected a few underlying pathological changes; there might still be only one disease.

The localisation of pathology

For the existence of distinct diseases to be firmly established, it was necessary for medical science to go inside the body and identify the precise spot where this or that disease was located. The increasing reductionism of biological science had its medical counterpart in the increasing *localisation of pathology*. However, before any of this could happen, medical scientists had first to learn what the normal workings of the body were like.

☐ Why did studies of the normal body have to come first?
■ Because it was only when the normal had been identified that the abnormal, and particularly the diseased or pathological state, could be recognised.

The exploration of the normal interior workings of the body was begun early in the Renaissance by anatomists in Italian universities. By 1543, Andreas Vesalius (1514–64) (see Figure 2.4), a Belgian physician working in Padua, was able to make a fundamental challenge to the classical tradition by showing that there were major errors in the anatomy established nearly 1 500 years before by Galen. The slow and painstaking work of dissection and description was conducted in every European country during the period but was, as we have seen, predominantly an Italian tradition, one that continued for several hundred years and provided a second essential observational base besides that given by purely clinical description. For once the anatomy of the normal body had been established, it provided the basis for the description of pathology, the study of diseased tissue.

The Italian anatomical tradition reached its culmination in the work of Giovanni Batista Morgagni (1682–1771). In Sydenham's day, in the mid-seventeenth century, clinical and post-mortem observation were separate fields of inquiry usually conducted by different people. Whereas one scholar worked on the minute description of symptoms quite unrelated to any internal bodily changes, another described pathological changes (lesions) without relating them to any particular symptoms. The clinician might describe 'consumption', a cluster of symptoms which involved coughing and fever; the pathologist, working at the dissecting table, might examine 'tubercules', small nodules in the lungs. Only when the two observations were put together would real advance be made. By the mid-eighteenth century there had been several such attempts to relate clinical and pathological findings, but it was Morgagni, in 1761 after fifty years of research, who best established the importance of combining the two methods. Not only did he relate pathology and clinical observation, but he seems to have realised that in any particular case this new intimacy should occur only *after* each side had conducted their own independent investigation of the disease.

☐ What is the scientific advantage of pathologists being allowed to read the clinician's report only *after* they have conducted a post-mortem?
■ Pathologists who have read the clinician's conclusions before the post-mortem already 'know' what they are looking for, and may both see what is not there and ignore many other important matters. Only if clinical and pathological observation are done independently, or *blind* as it is known, can the pathologist's work act as a systematic check on the physician's speculation about the cause of the disease.

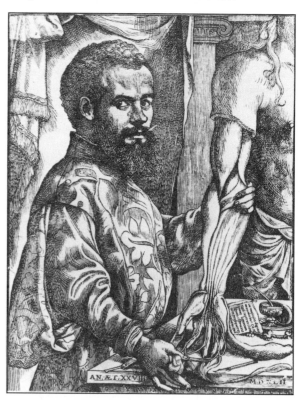

Figure 2.4 Andreas Vesalius.

This principle was of enormous importance. Here at last was a method to deflate theoretical enthusiasm and it remains a fundamental principle in medical research and practice. However, although it was the Italians who first brought clinical and pathological research together, it was in Paris in the early nineteenth century that the real power of this combination was demonstrated. The enormous hospital system that had been developed there enabled post-mortem and clinical investigation to be conducted for the first time on a massive scale. Large numbers of new diagnostic classifications were quickly made. To give a classic example, René Laennec (1781–1826) studied 167 clinical cases and autopsies in his work on 'pthisis', published in 1825. This at last brought together the clinical symptoms of consumption and the pathological findings of tubercles, thus identifying a new disease entity, tuberculosis, as the basis of three conditions previously considered to be independent: consumption, scrofula, and lupus (a skin condition).

The French school of pathology made further contributions besides that of systematic comparison and the study of very large numbers of cases. Morgagni had shown decisively that disease could be localised in organs. Now, in France, the detailed investigation of the anatomy of tissue was begun. At the same time, many sorts of new technology, such as the stethoscope (invented by Laennec), were introduced. Clinical and pathological observations were simultaneously improved by technological advance. However, although the French introduced some of this new technology, their use of it was limited compared with that by the new German school of medical research. For Germans now took the lead in medical advance, basing their work on a vastly improved microscope. The Dutch scientist Anthony van Leeuwenhoek (1632–1723) had produced a single-lens microscope over 100 years previously but its use was limited. A series of technical advances in the 1830s produced a compound microscope with increased powers of magnification (more than $500\times$ compared with $150\times$ previously). With the advent of the compound microscope researchers could study the individual cells of animal tissues. Johannes Müller (1801–58) developed the view that the cell was the basic unit of all living organisms, and Rudolf Virchow (1812–1902) then applied these techniques systematically to medical matters. With Virchow, the site of disease moved to the cells; the site of scientific advance from the wards and dissecting rooms to the laboratories. Virchow's own discoveries were wide-ranging, but his most crucial work was to demonstrate that particular diseases were accompanied by characteristic changes in cell structure and function. As such, he at last threw a little light on the nature of cancer.

Let us consider just one development in a little more detail, the way in which the improved microscope permitted the systematic identification of microorganisms. In the seventeenth century, van Leeuwenhoek had demonstrated their existence and the eighteenth century had seen a well-developed 'germ theory' of infectious diseases, though it was not widely accepted. However, only in the nineteenth century were microscopes and experimental techniques sufficiently advanced to show that germ theory was correct and older theories wrong.

There were several key steps in showing how microorganisms could cause disease. The first takes us, for a moment, from the history of medical science into the history of the brewing industry. There had been a long debate over the role of microorganisms in fermentation, the process in which sugar is turned into alcohol. Were yeast cells the *cause* of fermentation or were they merely a by-product, a life-form actually generated by the chemical process? A French biologist, Louis Pasteur (1822–95), showed conclusively, by careful experimental procedure, that if liquids were made sterile by boiling, and kept sterile thereafter, no microorganisms appeared and no fermentation ensued. So microorganisms were a cause of biological change rather than a mere effect. However, the implications of these findings had still to be applied to medicine. New techniques in microscopy and culturing had first to be developed. In 1876, nearly twenty years later, a German scientist, Robert Koch (1843–1910), proved for the first time that microorganisms could cause disease; that a specific bacterium caused a specific disease — anthrax. Pasteur himself reached the same result almost simultaneously. Further discoveries followed rapidly (Figure 2.5). Koch isolated the cholera and tuberculosis bacilli, the latter

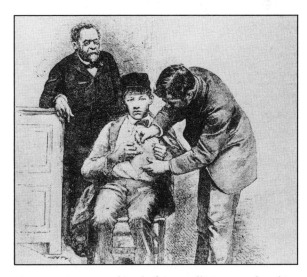

Figure 2.5 Pasteur watching the first test of his new cure for rabies.

responsible for one-seventh of the deaths from all known causes at that time. Further key discoveries were the bacteria responsible for diphtheria (1883), typhoid (1884), tetanus (1884) and bubonic plague (1894).

The search for cures

The French writer Voltaire (1694–1778) once defined doctors as people who poured medicine, of which they knew little, into bodies of which they knew nothing. For all Voltaire's scorn, doctors were beginning to learn something useful about medicines by the end of the eighteenth century. The traditional pharmacy, or 'materia medica', contained a diverse array of drugs and potions. Here, for example, is a seventeenth-century recipe for 'oil of swallows', a cure for 'shrunken sinews':

> Take young swallows out of their nests, by number twelve; rosemary tips, bay leaves, lavender tops, strawberry leaves, of each a handful; cut off the long feathers of the swallows, wings and tails, put them into a stone mortar and lay the herbs upon them and beat them all to pieces, guts, feathers, bones and all
> .... (quoted in Turner, 1958, p.25)

Not every doctor, however, believed that young swallows cured old sinews; many were now sceptical of the traditional remedies and, during the next two or three hundred years, the simple method of trial and error was applied to large numbers of treatments, many of which subsequently disappeared from medical practice. Trial and error also showed that just a few of these traditional treatments were, in fact, highly effective. Of these, the most spectacularly successful was cinchona bark, introduced from Peru in the Americas in the mid-seventeenth century and held by some sceptical physicians to be of more comfort to the sick than all the elaborate medical 'systems' put together. This drug, from which quinine (still a major treatment for malaria) was later isolated, made a profound impression on many doctors. It seemed strange that the 'untutored heathen' could advance medicine more than university trained physicians. Nevertheless, it offered hope that there were other remedies 'out there' waiting to be tried. Closer to home, there were major successes with local folk remedies by the end of the eighteenth century. The heart drug, digitalis, made from the foxglove, was introduced into the pharmacy. It, like the notion that fresh food could prevent scurvy, was originally a popular remedy.

But all in all, scientific medicine still had very few cures. As a result, by the beginning of the nineteenth century, some doctors, particularly in France, were openly sceptical of almost every form of medical therapy and concentrated their efforts instead on basic research, on description not treatment. Doctors like Laennec who undertook the

massive work of linking post-mortems to clinical observation took a bleak view of the possibility of medicine curing most of their patients; so bleak that their opinion was known as *therapeutic nihilism*. This extreme scepticism did, however, lead to major developments in improving the method of trial and error. The classic work here was a detailed study, published in 1835, of the effectiveness of blood-letting, the basic remedy in the humoral tradition. Pierre Louis' (1787–1872) method differed from previous studies of treatment in that he gathered a large number of similar cases, some of whom had had the therapy and others who had not, and applied statistical methods to the results. Blood-letting turned out to be of uncertain value. The same technique was quickly tried on new as well as old systems of therapy. Homeopathy did not work either. Physicians had been led astray through relying on their unsystematic personal impressions, though some clung on to blood-letting till the beginning of this century and homeopathy is still popular with the British Royal Family.

To the therapeutic nihilists, nature itself was the best cure. Most often, so they argued, there was no need to intervene, for most disease was *self-limiting*; it ran its natural course and then ended. Intervention might do more harm than good. Jacob Bigelow, a Harvard physician, argued in 1835 that it was 'the unbiased opinion of most medical men of sound judgement and long experience ... [that] ... the amount of death and disaster in the world would be less, if all disease were left to itself.' Not everyone found this an acceptable position, however great their scepticism about contemporary medical practice. By mid-century, some German pathologists raised a new cry: 'Wir wollen heilen, und nicht klassifizieren.' ('We want to heal, not classify.') To them, the overwhelming emphasis of the French school on post-mortems was too detached from human suffering. Medicine had to offer cures as well as understanding.

New cures were, however, being developed precisely at this point. For example, armed with new knowledge of the precise sites of diseases, and taking a key role in the discovery of such sites, surgeons now operated to remove the diseased tissue. In 1800, an old complaint — acute pain in the lower side — was treated by physicians who used purging or, somewhat later, morphine. Shortly after this date, the local pathology of 'appendicitis' was described and clear cases of rupture were found on post-mortem. Now that a surgeon could intervene, Henry Hancock from London performed the first appendicectomy in 1848. The new localisation of pathology was thus matched by a *localisation of therapy*.

For this operation and most others to become routine, two further developments were necessary. The first was the development of anaesthetics, itself a product of the new chemistry. It was introduced to medical practice by two American dentists, Stanley Wells (1815–48) and Horace Morton (1819–68) in the 1840s, and spread rapidly throughout medicine. The second development was some way of preventing the infection of the surgical wound that had hitherto been the most powerful bar to most types of surgery. Joseph Lister (1827–1912), a Glasgow surgeon, was referred by a chemist to Pasteur's initial work on bacteria and applied the results to surgery. He used carbolic acid to combat wound infection with dramatic results (see Figure 2.6). From 1864 to 1866, Lister performed 35 amputations, with fatal consequences in 16 cases. From 1867 to 1869, using antiseptic techniques, only 6 patients died out of 40.

Learning to copy Lister took time; carrying out anti-septic procedures demanded a strictness — an 'antiseptic conscience' as it came to be known — that many surgeons could not at first appreciate. However, by the end of the century, the new techniques enabled the most extra-ordinary growth in surgical practice. In 1899, a report by William Mayo of Minnesota on 105 gall-bladder opera-tions was rejected by a prominent medical journal because the total was thought implausible; five years later Mayo had an article in the same journal describing the results of 1 000 such operations.

Just as chemistry helped to revolutionise surgery, so it was applied with equally dramatic effect to the pharmacy. To begin with, work concentrated on isolating the active ingredients from the more successful traditional recipes. Morphine was isolated from opium in 1804, quinine from cinchona bark in 1822; both by French chemists. Special studies were also made of the old emetics and purgatives

such as epsom and glauber salts. Some biologists studied the body's chemistry. Of these, the most famous was another Frenchman, Claude Bernard (1813–96). Using detailed experiments with animals, Bernard showed that poisons acted upon particular parts of the organism, not upon the body as a whole. Carbon monoxide, for example, acted directly upon the haemoglobin* of the red blood cells.

Such findings were important for therapy because Bernard was able to show that remedies also acted in the same fashion. Once the precise locale in which a drug operated was known, it could be used far more precisely. From pharmacy, the preparation and dispensing of drugs, there now developed pharmacology, the science of the action of such drugs upon the body. The basis of modern pharmacology, indeed the modern drug industry, was laid in 1902 by the German biochemist, Paul Ehrlich (1854–1915), who was working with a group of German and Japanese organic chemists. They tried to create a 'magic bullet', an entirely synthetic drug that was aimed to hit the precise spot where a disease was located, destroying it but leaving the rest of the body unharmed.

Syphilis was the first disease to be treated by the new techniques developed by Ehrlich. It was at that time a wide-spread and much feared disease, whose traditional treatment, mercury, had highly adverse side-effects. Ehrlich's earlier work had shown, to his surprise, that certain dyes stained specific tissues, leaving all other others unaffected. He wondered whether other compounds might be targeted specifically against the microorganisms that threatened the body's health, not just to stain them, but to kill them.

It had already been shown that arsenic would kill certain tiny parasites, trypanosomes, that caused a disease of horses. Ehrlich injected these parasites into mice, with invariably fatal effects, and then tried to cure them with various arsenical compounds. He and his team patiently developed and tested hundreds of different compounds. The six-hundred-and-sixth experiment worked. Since the trypanosomes were very similar to the newly identified cause of syphilis, Ehrlich injected the new drug, 'Salvarsan', into a syphilitic rabbit which recovered almost immediate-ly. Trials upon human patients were begun in Berlin in 1910, also with dramatic results. Patients whose vocal chords were so affected by syphilitic lesions that they could hardly speak had their voices back within a few days.

Given the theories of disease, traditional medicine had relied on panaceas, or cure-alls, drugs which aimed to treat every form of disease. The techniques used to develop 'Salvarsan' offered something different. Not since quinine

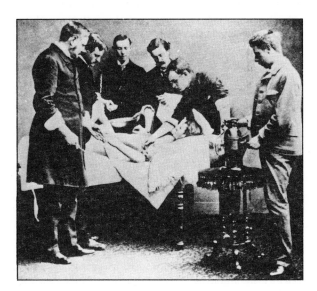

Figure 2.6 Lister's carbolic spray c.1870.

* The iron-containing pigment that has a high affinity for oxygen and hence acts as a carrier for it in the blood.

was first isolated from cinchona bark had there been such a powerful 'specific'; moreover, 'Salvarsan', unlike quinine, had been produced almost entirely in the laboratory. The twentieth century has seen many more such synthetic drugs, of which the most famous were the sulphonamides in the 1930s and penicillin in the 1940s, drugs which have dramatically lowered mortality from a whole range of infections.

Return of the sickman

Our principal theme has been the progressive localisation of disease by scientific methods and the development of effective remedies, first by trial and error, and later by more rigorous experiment. Traditional medical theory had held there to be merely one disease which had effects throughout the entire body of the individual. At the same time, as you may recall, it was thought that each individual experienced the disease differently and the doctor's job was to pay close attention to the particular set of balances and imbalances that were manifested in a particular patient, modifying the balance through purges, bleeding, alcohol, etc. Throughout, doctors kept their focus on the individual, the 'sickman'.

    ☐   In what ways did the new scientific medicine change this picture?
    ■   It showed that there were many diseases, not just one; such diseases were located at precise sites within the body; many traditional remedies, such as bleeding, were shown by careful trials to have no beneficial effect and might even be harmful; effective therapies for some diseases could be targeted at precise sites within the body; to understand both disease and therapy, it was shown to be essential to study large numbers of cases, not just particular individuals.

However, although the new discoveries were a major shift from the views of academic medicine, there is also an important respect in which many of the new discoveries led to a restatement, though in very different terms, of something resembling the more traditional view of health and disease. Let us begin by considering 'germ theory', one of the great triumphs of the new school of localised pathology. Pasteur and Koch might have shown that bacteria existed, but they had still left much unanswered. If some people died from the effects of bacteria, why did others survive? One nineteenth-century opponent of germ theory drank a whole glassful of cholera bacilli — and suffered no ill effects. Perhaps some people were naturally resistant to the disease, were blessed with a 'strong *constitution*' — an old term which had disappeared from scientific medicine, though it had been retained by the folk tradition. More support for theories of the importance of the individual constitution came in the late nineteenth century from the new science of genetics. Resistance or vulnerability to disease turned out to be, in some cases at least, partly a matter of heredity. A strong or weak constitution could be inherited from one's parents.

The late nineteenth century also saw a revival of some of the old humoral theories. New findings from biochemistry re-emphasised the importance of bodily fluids, for example bacterial infection of the blood (septicaemia) was found to be a humoral condition involving the whole body. Claude Bernard was, once again, the pioneering figure. In a further series of studies, this time of the process of digestion, he showed, for example, that sugar — in the form of glycogen — was stored in the muscles and liver, and that a relatively constant amount was always present in the blood; a discovery which paved the way for later studies in diabetes.

Such work led to the creation of another new specialism, that of endocrinology. By the end of the nineteenth century, it had been found that the pituitary, thyroid and adrenal glands produce 'hormones', chemical substances which are secreted directly into the bloodstream and which regulate the operation or development of other parts of the body. Balance theories had some truth after all. Indeed, Bernard argued that the health of the individual depended upon a constant interplay between internal and external environments. Every animal or plant, in order to survive, had both to resist the onslaughts of its environment and to maintain itself in a state of internal equilibrium, or *homeostasis*. The body's chemistry worked properly only within fairly narrow limits.

Such re-statements in a new form of traditional theories of bodily harmony and individual constitution led to the academic revival of some old interests. By the end of the nineteenth century, some German physicians were trying to study their patients' psychology as well as their physiology; the sickman was starting to return. There was also a revival of some traditional forms of cure. The belief that disease was more likely if someone was 'run down' was restated. Treatment now came to include methods for improving the patient's 'general condition'; diet, rest, exercise — all these received a new importance. Such methods had never, in fact, quite gone away. They had always been a standard part of much common sense and some ordinary medical practice. However, they were now coming at last to be incorporated within professional medicine. The process of incorporation, however, was and still is extremely slow. Breaking the body down into millions of tiny components has taken several hundred years of careful research and the process is by no means complete. Learning how to put the pieces together again will take just as long, or even longer, for new pieces are still being found all the time.

Pernicious anaemia: a case study

Having quickly reviewed some of the key trends in the development of modern biomedical science, let us illustrate some of the main points in more concrete detail by considering a classic scientific detective story — the slow unravelling of the mysteries of pernicous anaemia. Irvine Loudon, a general practitioner (GP) and historian of general practice, has reviewed this subject in a specially commissioned article. Turn now to Part 1, Section 1.6 of the Course Reader*. When you have finished Loudon's article, answer the following questions.

☐ Montaigne, in the passage criticising the practice of sixteenth-century medicine quoted earlier, stressed the complexity of nature. What features of the pernicious anaemia story illustrate this complexity?

■ Loudon points to the misleading clue of hydro-chloric acid; the fact that the disease involves both intrinsic and extrinsic factors; that it is a problem of the stomach and not of the blood; and, finally, the counter-intuitive notion that it may well be due to the body attacking itself, an auto-immune disease.

☐ What methods and circumstances have helped doctors and scientists to unravel the causes of pernicious anaemia and to treat it successfully?

■ Loudon mentions the following: clinical observa-tion; post-mortem findings; experiments; animal research; and, finally, chance (though, as Pasteur once said, 'Chance only favours the prepared mind').

The new faith

By 1870, the new science had set a pattern of thought and practice that was to dominate medicine during the next 100 years. There were, of course, enormous changes over that period but most of them involved the elaboration and putting into detailed practice of ideas that had already been established. The new disciplines, methods and reforms formed a solid basis from which scientific medicine could continue its advance. That advance, however, took place, at least initially, in the face of considerable public scepticism about medicine, for the therapeutic nihilism of the early nineteenth century had had serious effects on public confidence. If leading medical scientists confessed that medicine had very few cures to offer the sick, what was the average patient to make of it all? And the zeal of the medical reformers cast grave doubts on the most respectable parts of the profession. In 1823, for example, a new medical journal, *The Lancet*, had mounted a furious assault against many of the leading authorities of the day. No holds were barred. In one issue, its editor, Thomas Wakley, called the Royal College of Surgeons 'this sink of

infamy and corruption, this receptacle of all that is avaricious, base, worthless, and detestable in the surgical profession.'

Not only was there open warfare between many members of the profession, but most physicians were helpless in face of such scourges as the cholera epidemic of 1831 and, given the doctrines of therapeutic nihilism, many felt that nothing could be done. Much of the effective action was taken not by doctors, but by statisticians and engineers who both saw the need for and were more ready to deal with social reforms such as proper sewers, clean water and better housing to combat disease. Indeed, when the government created the first Board of Health in 1848, no physician was appointed to it. Academically trained doctors were temporarily at a very low ebb. An editorial in *The Times* in 1856 commented, 'The President of the Royal College of Physicians is so nearly on a par with the meanest herbalist. The result of the longest, most profound medical experience is so often a discussion of the worthlessness of medicine.'

All this was to change. The new advances in bacteriology, helped by Pasteur's flair as a publicist, gained scientific medicine immense credit. At Melun in France in 1881, Pasteur arranged a public demonstration of the effectiveness of his new anthrax vaccine. Every sheep not vaccinated by him succumbed to the injection of anthrax bacilli and did so in the presence of awed farmers, vets and reporters. Paul de Kruif, author of a popular history of bacteriology, described the impact thus:

> The world received this news and waited, confusedly believing that Pasteur was a kind of Messiah who was going to lift from men the burden of all suffering. France went wild and called him her greatest son and conferred on him the Grand Cordon of the Legion of Honour. Agricultural societies, horse doctors, poor farmers . . . all these sent telegrams begging him for thousands of doses of the life-giving vaccine. (quoted in Shryock, 1979, p.337)

The era of the 'medical miracle', of popular faith in the triumph of scientific medicine, had begun. As scientific advance gathered speed, so that faith slowly increased over the next 75 years to reach a climax in the years immediately following the Second World War. Scenes even more extravagant than those which had greeted Pasteur were to follow the development of a vaccine for polio. Whereas other infectious diseases had retreated, polio, an ancient disease (see Figure 2.7), had actually increased in incidence. Above all, its main target was children. In 1952, more American children died of polio than of any other infectious disease, and the polio charity, The March of Dimes, raised more money than any other medical charity of the period. When a vaccine was eventually developed,

* Black, Nick, *et al.* (eds) (1984) *Health and Disease: A Reader*, The Open University Press. (The Course Reader)

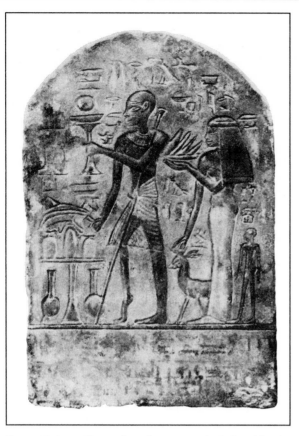

Figure 2.7 A sacrifice to Ishtar, the Egyptian God of Health. The priest's leg is deformed by childhood poliomyelitis.

millions of people took part as subjects in the clinical trials that were held in 1954. On 12 April 1955, scientists at the University of Michigan announced that the vaccine worked. Richard Carter, the biographer of Jonas Salk, the main creator of the vaccine, commented thus:

> more than a scientific achievement, the vaccine was a folk victory. People observed moments of silence, rang bells, honked horns, blew factory whistles, fired salutes, kept their traffic lights red in brief periods of tribute, took the rest of the day off, closed their schools or convoked assemblies therein, drank toasts, hugged children, attended church, smiled at children, forgave enemies. (quoted in Starr, 1982, p.347).

Paul Starr, an American sociologist, comments thus:

> The magic of science and money had worked. And if polio could be prevented, America had reasons to think that cancer and heart disease and mental illness could be stopped too. Who knew how long human

life might be extended? Medical research might offer passage to immortality. Between 1955 and 1960, unswerving congressional support pushed up the NIH (National Institutes of Health) budget from $81 million to $400 million. (Starr, 1982, p.347)

Whig history; a postscript

So that was the rise of biomedical science. Exciting stuff. But exactly how much truth is there in the story? Is modern medicine really quite so wonderful? Just as the first half of the nineteenth century saw a wave of criticism of medicine, so once again the nature and adequacy of medical knowledge has come under close scrutiny. The confident assumption of a huge leap forward in human understanding has been challenged. The particular relevance of the biological sciences to medical progress has been questioned and, as before, there are therapeutic nihilists both within and without the medical profession.

But before we consider the actual criticisms, a brief word about the nature of the history you have just read. Most of this chapter is written in a style which English-speaking historians call *Whig history*. The Whigs were the old version of the Liberal Party; they dominated British politics for almost the whole of the eighteenth century, while the Tories sulked in opposition. The Whigs were in power at the time when Britain itself grew to be the most powerful country in the world. So Whig history is the sort of history that is written by the confident and the successful. It is a story full of heroes performing valiant deeds against great odds and, despite the many setbacks on the road, their efforts are eventually crowned with triumph. This Whig view of history is a standard way of approaching the subject — any nation, any occupation, any faction that has ever met with success writes its own Whig history. Since medicine has met with a great deal of success, there is an awful lot of Whig history in the myriad of books, films and television programmes about medicine.

This way of writing history simply assumes that scientific biomedicine is a good thing; that it really has made dramatic progress in combating disease — as Bacon, Boerhaave and Paracelsus hoped it would. The precise extent of the progress that has occurred, the effectiveness of the new techniques, are left unexamined. As we shall see in Chapter 3, these are serious questions. There are other omissions. By and large, the historical context in which scientific innovation came about has been excluded. We have focused on Sydenham, Morgagni and Bernard but removed them from the world in which they actually lived; a world which was very different from today's. We have selected the bits we like and ignored those matters which now seem bizarre, foolish, cruel or simply different. By focusing so much on particular individuals, we have ignored not only the thousands upon thousands of other researchers, but also the wider social, economic and political factors which shaped the time and the thoughts of those who created scientific medicine.

If the past is judged solely from the standpoint of a triumphant present, there is a terrible temptation to spot forerunners, ancestors, harbingers of good news, people who were ahead of their time and who, like John the Baptist crying in the wilderness, had the essential truth, even though no one listened. The next step is easy. Once the chosen few have been assembled, the historian makes links between them and constructs a neat pattern in which the word is passed on, like a baton in a relay race, until the winner breasts the tape and is acclaimed by the multitude.

What is wrong with having heroes? Everyone likes to have them. Why should not doctors and biologists be allowed a few of their own, even at the cost of a little historical inaccuracy? At one level, this is harmless. But such inaccuracy can have serious consequences, for in studying history we study ourselves. We read the past in order to understand the present better. History can be used either to celebrate or to criticise contemporary life. Thus, a Whig history of scientific medicine is more than a history. It is also a justification of the claims of contemporary medicine; indeed, it is a central means by which contem-porary medical authority is bolstered. And, if some of the claims of contemporary medical science are wrong, history can also serve as propaganda.

There is therefore a need for more sceptical historians to investigate the bits that the Whig historians leave out. Of course, these sceptics are also likely to be biased, albeit in another direction. Those historians of medicine who are critical of some aspects of contemporary medicine are likely to reflect this in their own work. No historian can escape the influence of the present. This does not mean that 'history is bunk', as Henry Ford once said. Out of the swirl of argument and counter-argument, new facts are discovered, new knowledge created, as each of the various sides — and there are many — uncovers new evidence to be used in the debate.

Using the historical case studies contained later in this book, we shall both extend and reconsider the assumption of continuous progress that was made in the predominantly Whig history of this chapter. For the moment, however, we turn in the next chapter to some anthropological reflections. We see what we may learn about medical knowledge if we take a *cross-cultural* as well as an historical view; if we look beyond Europe to the rest of the human world and all of its diversity of form and thought.

Objectives for Chapter 2

When you have studied this chapter, you should be able to:

2.1 Describe the importance for the development of medical science of empirical methods, of systematic observation and experiment, as opposed to purely armchair speculation.

2.2 Outline the following aspects of changing medical belief and knowledge: the development of localised therapy and pathology in place of the monistic theories and remedies of traditional medicine with their emphasis on the individual sickman, on humours, solids and balances; the bringing together of clinical and pathological observation, and the consequent develop-ment of disease classification; the eventual partial return to modified theories of individual constitution and internal balance or homeostasis.

2.3 Describe the doctrine of therapeutic nihilism.

2.4 Outline the various ways in which medical authority is created, the ways these have changed over the centuries, particularly the shift from a more personal to a more collective style, and the role of science in this.

2.5 Discuss both the Renaissance doctrine of scientific progress and the Whig theory of historical progress.

Questions for Chapter 2

1 (*Objective 2.1*) What beliefs of the new Renaissance science do the following quotations illustrate? (Descartes and Aristotle were two philosophers.)

'More exact divisions on measuring instruments are more important than all of Descartes, all of Aristotle.' Albrecht von Haller, eighteenth-century physiologist.

John Hunter, a famous eighteenth-century anatom-ist, once said to Edward Jenner, the man who discovered smallpox vaccine, 'Why think, my dear Jenner, why not try?'

2 (*Objective 2.2*) (a) 'All the lingering chronic diseases and infirmities that one witnesses are only owing to not having been purged in some previous diseases, such as fevers, colds, inflammations, measles, smallpox or lyings-in. The Hygeists make use of only one medicine [the Gamboge Pill] and it cures everything.' James Morrison, 1829, inventor of the Gamboge Pill or Universal Medicine (quoted in Haley, 1978, p.14).

What form of medical theory does this represent and why?

(b) 'After qualifying at the University of Orange, Sloane handed Sydenham an introductory letter recommending him as "a ripe scholar, a good botanist, a skilful anatomist". Whereupon Sydenham, assuming his most severe military manner [he had been a cavalry officer in the Cromwellian Army] is alleged to have remarked "This is all very fine, but it won't do — anatomy, botany. Nonsense, Sir! I know an old woman in Covent Garden who understands botany better, and as for my anatomy, my butcher can dissect a joint full as well. No young man, all this is stuff: you must go to the bedside, it is there alone you can learn disease."' (quoted in Dewhurst, 1966, p.48).

(i) Why was the work of disease classification ultimately to involve anatomy, despite Sydenham's protestations?

(ii) In what way did Sydenham's version of learning at the bedside differ from the bedside medicine of the medieval tradition of the sickman?

(c) 'La fixité du milieu intérieure est la condition essentielle de la vie libre.' ('The stability of the body's internal environment is the essential condition for a free and unrestricted life.') (Claude Bernard, 1813–96)

Bernard's doctrine of homeostasis represents in some ways a return to classical medical theories of balance and harmony. In what ways, however, does it differ?

3 (*Objective 2.3*) What did Oliver Wendell Holmes, a nineteenth-century American doctor, mean when he called therapeutic nihilism 'the nature-trusting heresy'?

4 (*Objective 2.4*) 'The Prince listened to the doctor with a frown, now and then giving a little cough. As a man who had seen something of life, and was neither a fool nor an invalid, he had no faith in doctors, and in his heart was furious at the whole farcical business, the more so as he was probably the only one who really understood the cause of Kitty's illness. "Jabbering magpie", he thought.' (*Anna Karenina*, Tolstoy, 1877)

This was written in the nineteenth century. List some of the ways in which doctors traditionally tried to establish their authority. Which key method would have been unlikely to work with the prince? In what ways do modern doctors have a different basis on which to rest their authority?

5 (*Objective 2.5*) (a) The biography of Jonas Salk, the man after whom the Salk vaccine against poliomyelitis was named, is entitled *Breakthrough: The Saga of Jonas Salk*. In what ways do the names of the book and of the vaccine illustrate a Whig theory of medical history?

(b) 'Antiquity deserveth that reverence, that men should make a stand thereupon and discover what is the best way, but when the discovery is well taken, then to make progression.' (Bacon, *The Advancement of Learning*, 1605, quoted in Quinton, 1980, pp.28–9)

What was new about this doctrine in medical science?

3
Popular beliefs in the age of science

During this chapter you will be referred to three articles in the Course Reader: René Dubos, 'Mirage of health' (Part 1, Section 1.1); Cecil Helman, 'Feed a cold, starve a fever' (Section 1.2); and Ivan Illich, 'Epidemics of modern medicine' (Part 3, Section 3.7).

One of the commonest themes in writings about scientific progress is that today is a new age, an age in which everything has changed. The present is labelled the computer age; thirty years ago was the atomic age and before that the ages of electricity and of steam. All these developments are of major significance. Can our medical knowledge, our health beliefs and practices have anything in common with non-literate people who use a stone-age technology, a way of life that was abandoned in Western Europe over 4000 years ago, or with a village of Mexican peasants? Medical anthropology can help us to answer this question and in doing so can help to throw light on ourselves.

We shall begin the comparison by looking at the health beliefs of one group of people, the Nacirema, who have been studied by the American anthropologist Horace Miner. Here is the text of his article 'Body ritual among the Nacirema' (Miner, 1956, pp.503–7).

The anthropologist has become so familiar with the diversity of ways in which different peoples behave in similar situations that he is not apt to be surprised by even the most exotic customs. In fact, if all of the logically possible combinations of behaviour have not been found somewhere in the world, he is apt to suspect that they must be present in some yet undescribed tribe. This point has, in fact, been expressed with respect to clan organization by Murdock.[1] In this light, the magical beliefs and practices of the Nacirema present such unusual aspects that it seems desirable to describe them as an example of the extremes to which human behaviour can go.

Professor Linton first brought the ritual of the Nacirema to the attention of anthropologists twenty years ago,[2] but the culture of this people is still very poorly understood. They are a North American group living in the territory between the Canadian Cree, the Yaqui and Tarahumare of Mexico, and the Carib and Arawak of the Antilles. Little is known of their origin, although tradition states that they came from the east. According to Nacirema mythology, their nation was originated by a culture hero, Notgnihsaw, who is otherwise known for two great feats of strength — the throwing of a piece of wampum across the river Pa-To-Mac and the chopping down of a cherry tree in which the Spirit of Truth resided.

Nacirema culture is characterized by a highly developed market economy which has evolved in a rich natural habitat. While much of the people's time is devoted to economic pursuits, a large part of the fruits of these labours and a considerable portion of the day are spent in ritual activity. The focus of this activity is the human body, the appearance and health of which loom as a dominant concern in the ethos of the people. While such a concern is certainly not unusual, its ceremonial aspects and associated philosophy are unique.

The fundamental belief underlying the whole system appears to be that the human body is ugly and that its natural tendency is to debility and disease. Incarcerated in such a body, man's only hope is to avert these characteristics through the use of the powerful influences of ritual and ceremony. Every household has one or more shrines devoted to this purpose. The more powerful individuals in the society have several shrines in their houses and, in fact, the opulence of a house is often referred to in terms of the number of such ritual centres it possesses. Most houses are of wattle and daub construction, but the shrine rooms of the more wealthy are walled with stone. Poorer families imitate the rich by applying pottery plaques to their shrine walls.

While each family has at least one such shrine, the rituals associated with it are not family ceremonies but are private and secret. The rites are normally only discussed with children, and then only during the period when they are being initiated into these mysteries. I was able, however, to establish sufficient *rapport* with the natives to examine these shrines and to have the rituals described to me.

The focal point of the shrine is a box or chest which is built into the wall. In this chest are kept the many charms and magical potions without which no native believes he could live. These preparations are secured from a variety of specialized practitioners. The most powerful of these are the medicine men, whose assistance must be rewarded with substantial gifts. However, the medicine men do not provide the curative potions for their clients, but decide what the ingredients should be and then write them down in an ancient and secret language. This writing is understood only by the medicine men and by the herbalists who, for another gift, provide the required charm.

The charm is not disposed of after it has served its purpose, but is placed in the charm-box of the household shrine. As these magical materials are specific for certain ills, and the real or imagined maladies of the people are many, the charm-box is usually full to overflowing. The magical packets are so numerous that people forget what their purposes were and fear to use them again. While the natives are very vague on this point, we can only assume that the idea in retaining all the old magical materials is that their presence in the charm-box, before which the body rituals are conducted, will in some way protect the worshipper.

Beneath the charm-box is a small font. Each day every member of the family, in succession, enters the shrine room, bows his head before the charm-box, mingles different sorts of holy water in the font, and proceeds with a brief rite of ablution. The holy waters are secured from the Water Temple of the community, where the priests conduct elaborate ceremonies to make the liquid ritually pure.

In the hierarchy of magical practitioners, and below the medicine men in prestige, are specialists whose designation is best translated 'holy-mouth-men'. The Nacirema have an almost pathological horror of and fascination with the mouth, the condition of which is believed to have a supernatural influence on all social relationships. Were it not for the rituals of the mouth, they believe that their teeth would fall out, their gums bleed, their jaws shrink, their friends desert them and their lovers reject them. They also believe that a strong relationship exists between oral and moral characteristics. For example, there is a ritual ablution of the mouth for children which is supposed to improve their moral fibre.

The daily body ritual performed by everyone includes a mouth-rite. Despite the fact that these people are so punctilious about care of the mouth, this rite involves a practice which strikes the uninitiated stranger as revolting. It was reported to me that the ritual consists of inserting a small bundle of hog hairs into the mouth, along with certain magical powders, and then moving the bundle in a highly formalized series of gestures.

In addition to the private mouth-rite, the people seek out a holy-mouth-man once or twice a year. These practitioners have an impressive set of paraphernalia, consisting of a variety of augers, awls, probes and prods. The use of these objects in the exorcism of the evils of the mouth involves almost unbelievable ritual torture of the client. The holy-mouth-man opens the client's mouth and, using the above mentioned tools, enlarges any holes which decay may have created in the teeth. Magical materials are put into these holes. If there are not naturally occurring holes in the teeth, large sections of one or more teeth are gouged out so that the supernatural substance can be applied. In the client's view, the purpose of these ministrations is to arrest decay and to draw friends. The extremely sacred and traditional character of the rite is evident in the fact that the natives return to the holy-mouth-men year after year, despite the fact that their teeth continue to decay.

It is to be hoped that, when a thorough study of the Nacirema is made, there will be careful inquiry into the personality structure of these people. One has but to watch the gleam in the eye of a holy-mouth-man, as he jabs an awl into an exposed nerve, to suspect that a certain amount of sadism is involved. If this can be established, a very interesting pattern emerges, for most of the population shows definite masochistic tendencies. It was to these that Professor Linton referred in discussing a distinctive part of the daily body ritual which is performed only by men. This part of the rite involves scraping and lacerating the surface of the face with a sharp instrument. Special women's rites are performed only four times during each lunar month, but what they lack in frequency is made up in barbarity. As part of this ceremony, women bake their heads in small ovens for about an hour. The theoretically interesting point is that what seems to be a preponderantly masochistic people have developed sadistic specialists.

The medicine men have an imposing temple, or *latipso*, in every community of any size. The more elaborate ceremonies required to treat very sick patients can only be performed at this temple. These ceremonies involve not only the thaumaturge but a permanent group of vestel maidens who move sedately about the temple chambers in distinctive costume and headdress.

The *latipso* ceremonies are so harsh that it is phenomenal that a fair proportion of the really sick natives who enter the temple ever recover. Small children whose indoctrination is still incomplete have been known to resist attempts to take them to the temple because 'that is where you go to die'. Despite this fact, sick adults are not only willing but eager to undergo the protracted ritual purification, if they can afford to do so. No matter how ill the supplicant or how grave the emergency, the guardians of many temples will not admit a client if he cannot give a rich gift to the custodian. Even after one has gained admission and survived the ceremonies, the guardians will not permit the neophyte to leave until he makes still another gift.

The supplicant entering the temple is first stripped of all his or her clothes. In everyday life the Nacirema avoids exposure of his body and its natural functions. Bathing and excretory acts are performed only in the secrecy of the household shrine, where they are ritualized as part of the body-rites. Psychological shock results from the fact that body secrecy is suddenly lost upon entry into the *latipso*. A man, whose own wife has never seen him in an excretory act, suddenly finds himself naked and assisted by a vestal maiden while he performs his natural functions into a sacred vessel. This sort of ceremonial treatment is necessitated by the fact that the excreta are used by a diviner to ascertain the course and nature of the client's sickness. Female clients, on the other hand, find their naked bodies are subjected to the scrutiny, manipulation and prodding of the medicine men.

Few supplicants in the temple are well enough to do anything but lie on their hard beds. The daily ceremonies, like the rites of the holy-mouth-men, involve discomfort and torture. With ritual precision, the vestals awaken their miserable charges each dawn and roll them about on their beds of pain while performing ablutions, in the formal movements of which the maidens are highly trained. At other times they insert magic wands in the supplicant's mouth or force him to eat substances which are supposed to be healing. From time to time the medicine men come to their clients and jab magically treated needles into their flesh. The fact that these temple ceremonies may not cure, and may even kill the neophyte, in no way decreases the people's faith in the medicine men.

There remains one other kind of practitioner, known as a 'listener'. This witch-doctor has the power to exorcise the devils that lodge in the heads of people who have been bewitched. The Nacirema believe that parents bewitch their own children. Mothers are particularly suspected of putting a curse on children while teaching them the secret body rituals. The counter-magic of the witch-doctor is unusual in its lack of ritual. The patient simply tells the 'listener' all his troubles and fears, beginning with the earliest difficulties he can remember. The memory displayed by the Nacirema in these exorcism sessions is truly remarkable. It is not uncommon for the patient to bemoan the rejection he felt upon being weaned as a babe, and a few individuals even see their troubles going back to the traumatic effects of their own birth.

In conclusion, mention must be made of certain practices which have their base in native aesthetics but which depend upon the pervasive aversion to the natural body and its functions. There are ritual fasts to make fat people thin and ceremonial feasts to make thin people fat. Still other rites are used to make women's breasts larger if they are small, and smaller if they are large. General dissatisfaction with breast shape is symbolized in the fact that the ideal form is virtually outside the range of human variation. A few women afflicted with almost inhuman hypermammary development are so idolized that they make a handsome living by simply going from village to village and permitting the natives to stare at them for a fee.

Reference has already been made to the fact the excretory functions are ritualized, routinized and relegated to secrecy. Natural reproductive functions are similarly distorted. Intercourse is taboo as a topic and scheduled as an act. Efforts are made to avoid pregnancy by the use of magical materials or by limiting intercourse to certain phases of the moon. Conception is actually very infrequent. When pregnant, women dress so as to hide their condition. Parturition takes place in secret, without friends or relatives to assist, and the majority of women do not nurse their infants.

Our review of the ritual life of Nacirema has certainly shown them to be a magic-ridden people. It is hard to understand how they have managed to exist so long under the burdens which they have imposed upon themselves. But even such exotic customs as these take on real meaning when they are viewed with the insight provided by Malinowski when he wrote:

> Looking from far and above, from our high places of safety in the developed civilization, it is easy to see all the crudity and irrelevance of magic. But without its power and guidance early man could not have mastered his practical difficulties as he has done, nor could man have advanced to the higher stages of civilization.[3]

1   GEORGE P. MURDOCK, *Social Structure*, Macmillan, New York, 1949, p.71.
2   RALPH LINTON, *The Study of Man*, Appleton-Century, New York, 1936, p.326.
3   BRONISLAW MALINOWSKI, *Magic, Science and Religion*, Free Press, Glencoe, 1948, p.70.

☐   Who are the Nacirema?

■   Nacirema is 'American' spelt backwards, in case you did not realise. Do not worry if you were taken in by this anthropologist's joke — lots of people are.

Yet, of course, it is more than a joke. The fact that Miner can describe a culture so close to ours and so familiar, yet fool us all, makes a telling point. For all the advance of medical science, we remain a lot closer to non-literate cultures than we normally like to think.

☐   What are the (a) shrines, (b) taboos, (c) ritual obsessions, and (d) holy-men that Miner suggests are central to American health-beliefs in the 1950s?

■   Your list should look something like this: (a) shrines — the medicine-cabinet, wash-basin, hospital; (b) taboos — nakedness, sex, birth, excretion; (c) ritual obsessions — washing, shaving, hair-style, brushing teeth, body-size, breast-size, injections; (d) holy-men — doctors, dentists, psychiatrists.

☐   If Miner were to write a similar article about Britain in the 1980s, what things might he omit and what might he add?

■   Some taboos seem to have lessened — sex, birth and nakedness, for example. But others have begun to emerge: 'healthy' eating — bran, yoghurt, less fatty food; and exercise — jogging, yoga, and so on. Optimal body- and breast-size have undergone several changes since the 1950s while the frantic concern with both has come under heavy attack. Finally, there has been a resurgence of a different type of holy-man — acupuncturists, herbalists and the like.

Comparing 1950s America with the health culture of non-literate peoples, or with that of present-day Britain, teaches us one valuable lesson: the precise content of the beliefs and practices may change but shrines, rituals, taboos and holy-men (or women) remain. In certain respects, almost all cultures seem to share a common approach to health and disease. Having said this, there are also some important differences. But before going on to these, we shall first consider some more ways in which very different societies share similar health beliefs and practices.

The concept of health

'*Health*' seems at first a very modern obsession. Messages about it greet us from cereal packets, and assault our ears almost every time we turn on the television or the radio. Health is a new craze. And yet, as the following quotations remind us, an interest in health is unlikely to be a new phenomenon.

> How necessary Health is to our Business and Happiness: And how requisite a strong Constitution, able to endure Hardships and Fatigue is to one that will make any Figure in the World, is too obvious to need any Proof. (John Locke, 1632–1704, English philosopher and doctor)

> I live very quiet and very retired. I am now laying in a Stock of Health for the next Campagne. I get up (wonderful to tell) at eight O'clock every morning and Bath every day in the sea. Dine at half-past four and go to bed regularly at eleven. I am certain this Style of life will prolong my health at least ten years. (Mrs Fitzherbert, the morganatic wife of the Prince Regent, writing from Brighton in the early nineteenth century)

In the 1930s people were equally obsessed with exercise, sun and 'natural' products. The 1860s saw a craze for 'healthy' exercise and sport which was even greater than the jogging boom of the 1970s. At a Liverpool meeting of the Athletic Society of Great Britain in 1867, its president, John Hulley, addressed his audience in the rhetoric of the times:

> Physical education is the great fact of the nineteenth century. All over the country athletic festivals are

being celebrated. They must convince every unbiased mind that we are entering upon a new phase of national development. May the time come soon when weakly misshapen men and sickly, hysterical women will be the exception and not the rule among the inhabitants of our towns and cities. (quoted in Haley, 1978, p.138)

However, though an interest in health is universal, not every age or society pursues the same route. The sea-bathing followed by Mrs Fitzherbert was a novelty at the time and sun-worshipping came even later — in a largely rural society to be tanned is the mark of peasantry, not aristocracy. Nevertheless, for all these differences, research suggests that there are some striking uniformities in the way health is customarily defined. The following account draws on three studies: one of elderly Aberdonians by a British sociologist, Rory Williams; another of middle-class Parisians by the French sociologist Claudine Herzlich; and a third of Mexican peasants, living in a remote mountain area in New Mexico and Colorado. This last study was conducted by two American anthropologists, Sam Schulman and Anne Smith.

Each of these studies looked at very different sorts of people. Yet, as we shall now see, they found some remarkable similarities in the way health was defined. In each of the three cultures the routine greeting between friends also conveyed a hidden potential inquiry as to the state of the other's health: 'How are you?/I'm fine'; 'Comment allez-vous?/Je suis bien'; 'Cómo Está?/Bueno y Sano'. So health was seen as important and fundamental to the rest of life. It was also defined in very similar ways. One basic meaning was that of a stock or reserve of strength. The Mexicans spoke of those who had such a stock as possessing 'sangre fuerte' (strong blood); the Aberdonians talked of others who had 'lost' their health, who were 'done', 'broken down', 'finished', 'cracked up' or 'washed out'. By contrast those who had had reserves of health could come through many bouts of illness unscathed. They had, in the same words as the medieval theory, a 'strong constitution'.

☐ What other meanings of health can you think of?
■ The two most basic alternatives to the concept of a stock of health are those of fitness to perform tasks and the negative definition where health simply means an absence of pain or disease.

The notion of health as fitness, as something which enabled a person to perform their daily tasks, was central to all three cultures. In the Mexican village, the healthy person was the hard-worker. When asked to define what they meant by a 'healthy woman', one of the Mexicans replied that she 'works outside as well as inside ... she does her

housework, washes windows, is mujerota, a busy woman, is never too tired to keep her house and children neat and clean'. Likewise, the French spoke of the importance of possessing a 'bon équilibre mental' with which you could 'affronter tous les problèmes'. And if someone were without health, whether mental or physical, they could no longer perform the daily round or enjoy their ordinary pleasures. An Aberdeen man, who was no longer fit for work and had given up golf because of his angina, explained that his doctor had thumped him in the chest and said, 'You hang up your boots!' Finally, the notion of 'health' also meant the absence of pain or disease; to be healthy was to feel healthy, something that in all three cultures could lead to paradoxes. A Mexican health worker complained: 'If a person is big and strong and has a good colour, even though he may have TB, the people do not believe he is ill. If a person has intense pain (e.g. a tooth abscess) and shows it, the people believe he is ill.'

There were also some differences. The Mexicans placed a special emphasis on whether or not one was 'robusto' (husky) or 'gordo' (chubby), whereas Parisians and Aberdonians did not, though until recently most Aberdonian mothers believed that fat babies were healthy babies. Further, whereas the Aberdonians saw disease as primarily physical and were suspicious of malingering and hypochondria, the Parisians were much concerned with psychosomatic illnesses ('nerves' to the Aberdonians), with fatigue and with the necessity for tonics and 'fortifiants' and 'anti-anémiques'. Nonetheless, each culture shared the same basic approach. Health was a matter of reserves of strength, of fitness for daily life and of the absence of pain and disease; it was a matter of having, doing, and being.

There may well be other universal elements in the way different cultures think about health. Some intriguing arguments have been presented by René Dubos, a French-American biologist who discovered one of the first antibiotics, gramicidin. Turn now to the Course Reader (Part 1, Section 1.1) and study the series of extracts taken from his book, *The Mirage of Health*. When you have done so, answer the following questions:

☐ What, according to Dubos, are universal human dreams about health?
■ (a) A belief in a *utopian or ideal state of health*, set either in the past or the future; (b) a belief that such a state involves both a return to nature and the achievement of balance or equilibrium with nature.
☐ Why is this utopian state of harmony with nature both impossible and undesirable, according to Dubos?
■ Human beings are so flexible that they can live in almost any environment; there is no one 'nature' to which they can adjust. Indeed, the capacity to explore and to create new environments is the essential human

characteristic. Thus, to define one way of life alone as healthy is a dictatorship, not a utopia. It would confine, not free, the human 'spirit'.

☐ What is the relationship between curative and preventive theories of health, according to Dubos?

■ On his account, every society contains both types of theory, though cultures oscillate in the importance which they place on them. The Greeks gradually came to favour Asclepius, the god of therapy, rather than Hygeia, the goddess of prevention; the Victorians, for a time, re-instated the importance of Hygeia.

Let us retrace our steps a little. So far, we have seen that there are some standard views of health shared by people living in very different times and places. Health is a matter of reserves of strength, of the ability to fulfil one's daily round, of the absence of pain and disease. There are also some common human dreams: of a utopian state of health, of a harmony with nature and within oneself. Likewise, there is general agreement that achieving health involves both prevention and cure. So, although contemporary industrial society may be very different from that of traditional China or the Mexican highlands, certain aspects of the way people view health seem much the same. However, there are also some important differences to be noted. Henry Sigerist, a German historian of medicine, argued that for some medieval Christians, sickness was a healthier state than health itself. For them:

> Disease is suffering and it is through disease that mankind is completed. Suffering is the friend of the soul. It develops spiritual strength. It turns the gaze of the human spirit towards eternity. Sickness has become the cross which the sick man carries following in the footsteps of Christ .... Disease must be completely suffered, for it was in the very fullness of suffering that a human soul found purification.
> (Sigerist, 1977, p.389)

☐ How does this view differ from that expressed by John Locke on p.24? (Turn back to see what Locke said if you need to.)

■ Locke's gaze was not directed towards eternity, but towards more immediately practical ambitions — making a Figure in this World rather than the Next. He therefore placed an entirely different value on health.

Locke's view of health seems likely to be the more common one, even in medieval times. Nevertheless, the example reminds us that people can have very different views of the matter. Note also that the words 'health' and 'healthy' can have a very wide application. Here, for example, is a quotation from the Anglican *Book of Common Prayer*: 'We have left undone those things which we ought to have done; and we have done those things which we ought not to have done; and there is no health in us.' Sin is here equated with disease. As this suggests, the terms 'health' and 'healthy' can be applied to every aspect of human life, depending on the values of the speaker; indeed, they may function simply as a way of praising anything one happens to like.

The sick role

It has just been argued that most people in most societies want to stay healthy and that they share fairly similar definitions of what health is — provided, that is, that we make allowance for the very different sorts of lives they lead or prefer. So far, however, we have looked mostly at individual definitions of health, but an individual's state of health is of interest to many other people besides that particular person.

☐ Why might other people have an interest in your health?

■ There are several reasons: they may care for you; or, in another meaning of the word, realise that if you are sick they will *have* to care for you; or they may rely on you to be healthy so that you can perform some social task which is of interest to them.

As a result, there is a bundle of social rights and duties which surround sickness and health; something which the American sociologist Talcott Parsons in 1951 termed the *sick role*. Parsons also pointed to one further aspect of the sick role which has not yet been mentioned; an aspect which is treated in the following extract from a play written by Oscar Wilde in the 1890s:

ALGERNON I am afraid Aunt Agatha, I shall have to give up the pleasure of dining with you tonight after all.

LADY BRACKNELL [*frowning*] I hope not, Algernon. It would put my table completely out. Your Uncle would have to dine upstairs. Fortunately, he is accustomed to that.

ALGERNON It is a great bore, and, I need hardly say, a terrible disappointment to me, but the fact is I have just had a telegram to say that my poor friend Bunbury is very ill again. [*Exchanges glances with Jack*] They seem to think I should be with him.

LADY BRACKNELL It is very strange. This Mr. Bunbury seems to suffer from curiously bad health.

ALGERNON Yes; poor Bunbury is a dreadful invalid.

LADY BRACKNELL Well, I must say, Algernon, that I think it is high time that Mr. Bunbury made up his mind whether he is going to live or to die. This shilly-shallying with the question is absurd. Nor do I in any way approve of the modern sympathy with invalids. I consider it morbid. Illness of any kind is hardly a thing to be encouraged in others. Health is the

primary duty of life. I am always telling that to your poor Uncle, but he never seems to take much notice — as far as any improvement in his ailment goes. I should be much obliged if you would ask Mr. Bunbury, from me, to be kind enough not to have a relapse on Saturday, for I rely on you to arrange my music for me.
(Wilde, 1954, p.262)

The invalid 'Bunbury' is a fiction, invented by Algernon as an *excuse* for getting out of various social obligations — such as dining at Aunt Agatha's. In other words, as Lady Bracknell hints, sickness as well as health can sometimes be of personal advantage. The sick may use illness to excuse themselves from ordinary social duties, as may their friends and relatives who have to care for them. On Parson's analysis, the wider society shared Lady Bracknell's view that 'illness of any kind is hardly a thing to be encouraged in others'. He argued, therefore, that individuals who were sick had a crucial right and a crucial obligation. On the one hand, they could *claim* the right to be excused from many of their normal social duties but, on the other hand, they were also obliged to seek and follow the medical advice of friends, relatives and healers, to obey 'doctor's orders'. They had, in other words, a duty to get better. To match this, other people have a complementary set of rights and responsibilities. Healers, relatives and friends have a duty to care for the sick but in return they have the right to check the claims of the sick person to be ill. Health and illness are, therefore, not simply biological states. They are also social roles whose occupants must on occasion prove that they really are well or ill.

☐ What examples of such proof can you think of in contemporary Britain?
■ Absence from work on the grounds of illness normally requires a sickness certificate from a doctor to be produced after a specified number of days. Those who are disabled and wish to claim a pension or social security benefit must likewise submit to medical examination. And school children who wish to be excused games on the grounds of illness must normally provide a note from their parents or their doctor.

Parsons argued that the sick role was not peculiar to our society, but was universal to all cultures. Without it, a society could not function, for everyone would be like Algernon — avoiding whatever they could on the grounds of illness. Some people have challenged this, arguing that Parsons' model applies only to the United States or to modern states with their huge bureaucracies, health insurance systems and social security benefits. However, work by American anthropologists suggests that Parsons may be right. Something like the sick role appears to exist in non-literate as well as industrialised societies. There are, however, some exceptions that need to be made. It is not clear how far the role applies to certain forms of chronic illness or handicap, whether mental or physical in nature. People who are blind cannot get better by following doctors' orders. Those who are chronically depressed cannot just 'pull themselves together', as some of their friends may urge. Nevertheless, such people are still subject to medical inspection, still obliged to show that they are making some kind of an effort to conform. Erving Goffman, another American sociologist, once noted that even the paralysed, lying immobile in iron lungs, were expected to wink to show they were keeping their spirits up, thus making themselves less of a burden to their attendants.

There is also another sort of exception. Not everyone, so it turns out, recognises the existence of disease and, if sickness is not recognised, there can be no sick role. Take the example of a modern Japanese sect called Tensho. The founder, Ogamisama, preaches that sickness is due to a spirit which acts only if a member has neglected their religious duty. 'If you discipline yourself hard enough, you will enter the world where there is no need of doctors or drugs.' (quoted in Lebra, 1977, p.412) Tensho members do not help the sick in case they too should catch the spirit causing the illness. When ill themselves they struggle to carry on as if they were healthy, for it is the sect's boast that only through Tensho can one avoid illness, and to appear sick would frighten potential converts. Thus, though the sick role seems to be found in all societies, not everyone in those societies may necessarily accept it. Tensho may represent an extreme but we all know people who deny almost every form of illness, both in themselves and in others, just as we know others who rush to embrace it.

Choosing a healer

We began this chapter by considering the way in which many ritual elements still survive in modern health practices, at least on one anthropologist's interpretation. We then noted how there are many important similarities between very different societies, both in the meanings that people give to health and in the set of rights and duties that surround sickness. Now we shall examine the way in which people in different cultures set about choosing a healer, a term that covers a great variety of people besides doctors.

☐ What different sorts of healers could people in nineteenth-century France turn to, according to Zeldin's description?
■ As well as the numerous doctors with their rival systems, he refers to 'a whole army of rival practitioners offering cheaper and sometimes more acceptable treatment: the urine healer ... the orviétan merchants

(the itinerant sellers of drugs), the sorcerers, the nuns, the priests, the old women, the midwives, the pharmacists', along with the bone-setters, 'clairvoyantes' (who distributed magical and herbal cures) and those who ran the holy places 'where every disease was cured by miracles'.

Now compare this with a description of the range of healers in a modern central African city, beginning with the sort of healer most of us will know best — doctors and nurses trained in Western medical science. These can be found in free government clinics and also in private surgeries with their own system of referral to hospital consultants. The private doctors cater to the wealthy. There are, however, a variety of other cheaper healers who belong instead to African medical traditions. (Note that one should not make too rigorous a distinction between the different types of healers.) In the market place, for example, there are herbalists who provide diagnosis and therapy for a fee. The most renowned of these itinerant practitioners have a big local reputation and receive payment only by result — gifts from satisfied patients. The most prestigious healers are sponsored by the main political parties, both sides gaining credit from the association. There are also 'diviners', healers who specialise in the diagnosis of witchcraft and sorcery and offer protection against these afflictions. These practitioners have to practise with care. Too public an accusation can lead to riots and judicial proceedings. Finally, there are healers who specialise in the treatment of those possessed by evil spirits. Such healers enter into a trance, become temporarily possessed themselves and thereby deliver the sufferer from their affliction.

This last form of therapy often takes place in the street outside the healer's house, and involves dancing, music and songs. It is a communal drama, almost a form of entertainment, through which the possessed are returned to the bosom of society.

☐ In what way do the patients of the herbalists display a shrewd empirical approach to medicine?
■ They pay only by result.

Many poorer Africans in fact find the Western system of payment baffling. What use is expensive private medicine, they ask, if your spouse comes out of hospital in an even worse state than when they went in? Note also that the variety of healers serve quite distinct purposes. People with infections or broken limbs go to Western-style healers if they can. The chronically sick or mad are taken to the diviners and those who specialise in spirit possession. Finally, men who are impotent or have problems at work and women wondering whether their husbands are unfaithful, or whether their pregnancy will go well this time: all these seek the herbalists' advice.

☐ In what way does this use of a range of healers resemble our own practice in British society? What other sorts of contemporary healer can you think of besides Western doctors?
■ There is now, as there has always been, an enormous range of healers who compete with or complement physicians and surgeons. There are osteopaths (much favoured by football clubs); homeopaths (used by the Royal Family); acupuncturists; Christian Scientists; health-food stores; and herbalists. (Even the political sponsorship of different herbalists has a kind of British parallel. The Conservative Party traditionally favours the doctors, the Labour Party the ancillary workers!)

Some methods, such as herbalism, are modern developments of old traditions. Others, such as osteopathy, homeopathy and chiropractic, are nineteenth-century medical systems which began as rivals to the academic medicine of their day and which still survive, unlike the doctrines of Brown or Broussais mentioned in Chapter 2. And yet other systems have been imported from classical traditions of medicine which developed separately from that of Europe — acupuncture is the most popular of these.

Since the period which Zeldin describes, academic medicine has come to control a far larger share of the medical market. Yet it is still very far from driving out all its competitors. 'Alternative' or 'complementary' medicine, as it now likes to be known, is in fact a major sector of health care in Western societies (see Table 3.1, but note that this table omits the traditional medical practices used by recent immigrant populations in the UK — such as Indian Ayurvedic medicine). Moreover, what is counted as 'quackery' by doctors in one country may sometimes be normal medical practice in another. Visiting a spa is a central part of German health care and is currently under revival in France, although no longer fashionable in the UK. Osteopaths are banned in some countries and welcomed in others. Homeopathy still has one or two posts in some British hospitals, has several hospitals for clinical training in France, and 70 000 registered practitioners in India. Some British general practitioners also practise acupuncture. There is no hard and fast line to be drawn between what counts as 'respectable' medical practice and its rivals. It all depends where you look. In conclusion, in nineteenth-century France and twentieth-century Africa and Britain, there is a range of healers with whom the sick may try their luck. Even in the heartlands of 'Western medicine', the academic tradition is far from exerting a total monopoly; indeed, the latest wave of therapeutic nihilism has been accompanied by a new interest in alternative medicine. The complexities of health and disease still leave plenty of scope for rivals to the scientific tradition.

Table 3.1 Number of complementary practitioners in the UK, 1980

Therapy	Medically qualified	Lay members in professional association	Lay practitioners not in professional association
acupuncture	160	508	250
chiropractic	1	140	400
herbalism	10	103	200
homeopathy	272	130	230
hypnotherapy	1 000	460	170
massage	350	1 150	1 500
naturopathy	5	115	106
osteopathy	202	650	150

(Fulder and Monro, 1981, p.35)

Science in the Stone Age?

Many of the comparisons made in this chapter are not, at least on second thoughts, particularly surprising. Most of you will know someone who has been to an alternative healer, or you may have been yourselves. And though the identity of the Nacirema may possibly have come as a shock, it is common to talk of medical 'rituals', of 'worshipping' science and so forth. This section, however, covers something that is rather more unusual: the possibility that some societies with a stone-age technology might well have had quite sophisticated anatomical and medical knowledge, might possibly have been in advance of some sixteenth-century European academic medicine. It is impossible now to be sure of these matters, for the traditional culture of the Aleuts, a hunting people living in islands off Alaska, was largely destroyed by the turn of this century. However, the American biological anthropologist William S. Laughlin, who has studied the modern Aleuts as well as the historical records of their contacts with more modern societies, has constructed a most provocative argument.

The Aleuts were primarily hunters who relied on what they could catch for most of their food, clothing and possessions. Intestines were made into anoraks, shirts and bags; stomachs were used as floats and storage containers; the pericardium (the sac which encloses the heart) was used as a water-container; and so on. Just about every part of the animals they killed and butchered found a practical use and everyone was expected to have some expertise in the dissection of the dead animals. As a consequence, the ordinary Aleut possessed (as many still do) the most extraordinarily rich anatomical vocabulary. Children who forgot the name for this or that tiny part of an animal could be laughed at.

☐ What sort of people in contemporary industrial society have this sort of knowledge?

■ Only doctors, vets, human biologists and possibly butchers and farm-workers.

But the Aleuts, according to Laughlin, went a good deal further than simple butchery. In addition to the anatomical knowledge gained from killing animals, the Aleuts conducted extensive medical inquiries. Sick animals eat and drink very little, so they copied this — most of their medical treatments were based on fasting and resting. They dissected dead human beings, both to find out why they had died and to further their knowledge of human anatomy. Comparative anatomy was practised on the sea-otter, which was chosen because of its physical and behavioural resemblance to human beings (it can use rocks as tools to crush shellfish). Finally, they had developed techniques for mummifying the body, both to preserve and to study it.

Here then was a highly sophisticated level of medical knowledge; possibly well in advance of European knowledge for a long time. Their surgery was, not surprisingly, quite advanced; so too may have been their theoretical knowledge of illness. A related people, the Tungus, are known to have held a kind of germ theory. They inferred the existence of microorganisms from the observation of worms in wounds that gradually grew large enough to be visible to the naked eye, reckoning from this that there must be other, very small worms that could not be seen and which must cause disease.

The traditional Aleut and Tungus cultures are now gone for ever; only dim remnants exist. The last dissection of a human being was witnessed by an old woman, over 90 years old, who died in the 1930s. The last dissection of a sea-otter took place in 1911, at which time hunting the sea-otter was banned by the United States government. We shall therefore never know how much the Aleuts knew. Laughlin himself suggests that their anatomical knowledge was in advance of Galen and that they were almost certainly aware of the circulation of the blood. He goes on to point out that, although cultures such as the Aleut and the Tungus were very rare by the nineteenth and twentieth centuries, their way of life was once a common one. Fifteen thousand years ago, in the last Ice Age, glaciers covered much of Europe and Asia. As we can tell from the cave paintings which date from this period and even earlier, some of the peoples who hunted the great herds of deer, rhinoceroses and mammoths had a highly sophisticated culture. Their anatomical and medical knowledge may well have matched their artistic skill.

The survival of traditional belief

Having quickly examined various ways in which contemporary health beliefs and practices have their counterpart in traditional, non-literate societies, let us consider this in more detail by looking at some of the beliefs of a group of people living in a North London suburb. This study was conducted by a general practitioner, Cecil Helman, who has also trained as an anthropologist. He takes an apparently banal subject, ordinary colds and fevers, but his conclusions are far from ordinary. Turn now to the Course Reader (Part 1, Section 1.2) and study the article by Helman. When you have finished, answer the following questions.

☐ In what way does the popular use of germ theory resemble the magical beliefs of the Africans discussed previously?

■ Helman points out that the way many of his patients describe 'germs' is very similar to the African belief in invisible malign spirits.

☐ In what ways is medical practice not based on science at all?

■ Cough medicine is useless and antibiotics, though freely prescribed, do not work against viruses.

☐ In the health beliefs of Helman's patients, fluids were very important, as was the classification of hot, cold, wet and dry. What is the name of this medical theory?

■ Humoral theory.

Studies such as Helman's are still highly exploratory. Social scientists are only just beginning to explore the health beliefs of contemporary societies in any depth. Nevertheless, here is at least some evidence that *popular beliefs* about health and disease are still shaped by traditional thought such as the older form of humoral theory and the theory of attack by malign spirits. Helman also suggests that popular belief is modified by new organisational and scientific developments. Nineteenth-century germ theory and the creation of the National Health Service have clearly had an effect. Nevertheless, while such innovations may influence popular thought, they do not appear to transform it completely.

Natural and supernatural

We began this chapter by noting that the assumption of constant progress, so central to the Whig theory of history, could be criticised in a number of crucial ways. Anthropological evidence suggests some surprising resemblances to many of our own health beliefs. Traditional beliefs can still be found in a North London suburb; Mexican peasants, Parisian city-dwellers and elderly Aberdonians all seem to share very similar definitions of health; a hunting people with a stone-age technology may well have possessed sophisticated anatomical and medical knowledge. The moral seems to be that, although Western medical science has been dramatically transformed since the Renaissance, many medical beliefs and practices have stayed much the same. However, this is not quite the whole story. There is one fundamental way in which medical beliefs have changed; a way at which so far we have only hinted. The place of religion and of the *supernatural* has radically altered. Helman suggests that traces of such theories are still to be found in the way his patients talked about germs, but these are merely fragments of what was once a powerful intellectual tradition, a way of thinking about disease which seems to have dominated our own and every other society. That tradition is illustrated in the following quotation from the Bible which describes the origin and course of a major epidemic in the time of King David, nearly 3 000 years ago:

Thus saith the Lord, 'Choose thee: Either three years famine; or to be destroyed before thy foes while the sword of thine enemies over taketh thee; or else, three days the sword of the Lord, even the pestilence in the land, and the angel of the Lord destroying throughout all the coasts of Israel.' And David said 'I am in a great straight; let me now fall into the hand of the Lord, for great are his mercies; but let me not fall into the hand of man.' So the Lord sent pestilence unto Israel; and there fell of Israel seventy thousand men. And God sent an angel into Jerusalem to destroy it: and as he was destroying, the Lord beheld, and he repented him of the evil, and said to the Angel that destroyed, 'It is enough, stay now thy hand.'
(I Chronicles 21: 11–15)

☐ The Bible's language is often hard and the stories strange. Re-read the passage carefully and consider the ways in which the Israelites' views differ from most modern religious beliefs as regards the following topics:
(a) the cause of plague;
(b) the relationship between human beings and God;
(c) God's character and attitude towards human beings.

■ (a) In most modern religious views, God does not cause plagues; those are instead the result of micro-organisms and social conditions.

(b) Human beings and God do not communicate in this fashion.

(c) God has a rather better character — he no longer commits evil. Human beings can commit evil, but it seems odd to talk of God in these terms.

Of course, some religious people today believe that God does intervene in this fashion in human affairs, but most people, whether religious or not, have a different view. Even religious people do not normally believe that they are in direct contact with the Almighty. In the past, some people who saw visions or even God himself were regarded as saints. Their modern equivalents may end up in a mental hospital.

Nor do most people believe that God is regularly interfering with human destiny: dishing out punishments and rewards as appropriate, or showering harmful bacilli on the unfaithful. Instead, we place a great gulf between God and ourselves; we live in the *natural realm*, God in quite another. And if we do not believe in a god at all, then there is only the natural realm and nothing beyond it. But for people in most societies until very recently, God, spirits, devils, fairies, all regularly intervened in human lives or were invoked by human collaborators such as witches and sorcerers, and were, it would seem, the principal cause of disease.

Table 3.2 illustrates the results from a study of the theories of disease-causation prevalent in a sample of 186 societies selected so as to represent a wider group of 1 300

Table 3.2 The distribution of theories of disease-causation in a sample of 186 societies

Theory	Total score
infection	32
stress	77
deterioration	28
accident	39
fate (e.g. astrological influence)	30
'ominous sense' (e.g. vision or dream)	37
'pollution' (e.g. by menstruating woman)	50
taboo violation	154
soul loss (soul leaves body)	34
malevolent spirit	331
sorcery (a technique available to anyone)	221
witchcraft (only performed by a special category of evil persons)	88

(data from Murdock, 1980, pp.11–5, 22–6)

societies on which anthropological information was available. The data were drawn from an American source, the Human Relations Area File. For fifty years information from most human cultures has been systematically collected in this file. George Murdock, the American anthropologist in charge of the project, and his assistants devised twelve different categories of disease-causation (or aetiology), four of them covering natural theories and eight of them concerned with supernatural causes. The data on the theories of illness in each society were checked for each category of disease-causation and ranked on a scale from 0 to 3 depending on the importance of that category in the society. All but a handful of the societies are non-literate peoples with a fairly low level of technology.

There are many problems in interpreting this table. Not all anthropologists would agree with the definitions that Murdock uses; it is uncertain how far the data on each society are adequate; scoring societies on a 0 to 3 scale is also difficult. But, if all these problems can be set aside, the data do suggest that supernatural theories of illness are of overwhelming importance in traditional non-literate cultures. Not all societies held to such theories. The Greek doctors of the fifth century BC who worked in Cos and Cnidus believed strongly in natural explanations. Here, for instance, is an extract from a Greek essay on epilepsy, traditionally known as the 'sacred disease':

I do not believe that the 'sacred disease' is any more divine or sacred than any other disease but, on the contrary, it has specific characteristics and a definite cause ... those who first called the disease 'sacred' were the sort of people we now call witch-doctors, faith-healers, quacks and charlatans. These are exactly the sort of people who pretend to be very pious and particularly wise. By invoking a divine element they were able to screen their own failure to give suitable treatment and called this a 'sacred' malady to conceal their ignorance of its nature .... (anon. 'The Sacred Disease' in Lloyd, 1978, pp.237–8)

But purely naturalistic views were probably comparatively rare, even in Greek society. It was only with the Reformation, the sixteenth-century revolt by the Protestants against the Catholic Church, that a systematic attack was made on magical beliefs and practices in Europe, and even then the tradition died hard. Until the seventeenth century, for example, the Pope's physician was also the Vatican astrologer. Eventually, however, the new science and the new social, political and economic world of which it was a part swept most of these beliefs away. Today only fragments remain; though in some vague and disorganised way they may still exert a powerful effect, as the articles by Miner and Helman suggest.

Empirical and magical

We have now come almost to the end of this review of health beliefs in our own and other societies. But before we move on to the final part of this chapter, we must first address an important conflict between different schools of anthropology. One school of anthropologists, of whom William S. Laughlin is a good example, are also trained in the natural sciences. According to them, those anthropologists who are trained only in social science are too ignorant of botany and anatomy to make any proper assessment of the accuracy of the medical and scientific knowledge of those whom they are studying. In consequence, they are far too ready to write off a culture's healing practices as simply based on *magic*. Laughlin, for example, argues that until very recently none of the people who had studied the Aleuts had the knowledge, the interest, or the time to capture the full details of what these people knew. Only specialists such as himself would be able to talk in detail with the Aleuts concerning their anatomical knowledge. He comments:

> the consistent underestimation of primitive's knowledge is a notorious and unfortunate fact ... apparently without exception, every fieldworker who has included such an investigation in his schedule has remarked that he was unable to exhaust the native's knowledge because of too little time, or because he himself lacked the necessary knowledge to record those things that the native informant wished to tell or show him. (Laughlin, 1977, p.261)

It may also be that anthropologists have been misled by the exotic. They may, perhaps, have ignored the more everyday health beliefs which were similar to their own and focused instead on the magical practices. It is strange, for example, that, according to the data gathered in the Human Relations Area File, so few cultures seem to believe that one of the reasons for disease is the body's deterioration over time. Perhaps this belief was simply too obvious for anthropologists to record.

However, the school of anthropologists trained in social science also has some powerful arguments. They point to the natural scientists' ignorance of social processes and argue that it is naïve to imagine that people in such cultures have, by trial and error, stumbled across a great range of modern drugs simply through the elaboration of herbal remedies. They point out the attractions of this view to traditional healers eager to gain the blessings of Western science. Moreover, although it is certainly true that cocaine reduces the feelings of pain and hunger felt by American Indians and that the mould used by gypsies on wounds may have contained penicillin, it is equally true that many of these herbs and other substances have been selected for quite different reasons and have been applied in ways that render them biochemically inert. They argue, for example, that the medieval use of the mandrake root was directly associated with its distinctly forked shape that resembles the human body — something which explains the tales of how it was supposed to scream when wrenched from the soil. Similarly, many charms, like rabbits' feet, are applied momentarily or worn as amulets, and some are burnt or drunk, not as drugs, but for the sympathetic or protective influence they are expected to have on the patient or wearer. Trace elements may explain the efficacy of some herbs, but this may have little relationship to a culture's medical theory. The classic exponent of this point of view is the British anthropologist E.E. Evans-Pritchard, who argued of the African people he had studied, 'Zande remedies are of an almost completely magical order.' (Evans-Pritchard, 1934, p.53)

The debate continues and will do so for some time. Just as the social anthropologists normally lack botanical or anatomical knowledge, so the biological anthropologists are often insensitive to the way in which a culture's medical theory is shaped by the complex beliefs and relationships of the societies of which they are a part. But there is also a sense in which the two approaches are complementary. It is perfectly plausible for a culture to find a drug by trial and error, and, simultaneously, to develop a magical theory of how it works. Moreover, as we shall now see, there is nothing unusual in possessing a range of therapies, only a few of which are actually effective. But before we do this, there is one more task.

> ☐ Go back to Laughlin's quote and see if you can identify another factor which may have biased anthropologists' accounts of behaviour in other cultures.
> ■ The use of the term 'primitive', which was standard in anthropology for a long time, suggests that this discipline, like many others, was permeated by a conscious or unconscious racism.

The effectiveness of Nacirema medical practice

We began this chapter with Horace Miner's satirical article about American health beliefs. He suggests that the medicine chests in American houses are filled with charms and magical potions, that hospital physicians are medicine-men, psychiatrists witch-doctors. What evidence is there for this? As we have just said, it is possible to have magical beliefs about an effective therapy. But satire such as Miner's will itself be more effective if it can be shown that the remedies do not work, that medicine's claims are simply claims.

> ☐ What arguments have you come across in this chapter to suggest that scientific medicine may not be as effective as it is sometimes made out to be?

■ Dubos argued that the reason for the disappearance of epidemic disease on a dramatic and fatal scale in the nineteenth century was due to sanitary reform rather than bacteriology. The new public health, with its emphasis on clean water, improved sewage disposal and better housing, was the real cause. And Helman suggested that, although all kinds of antibiotics were now available, they were often prescribed for diseases they could not treat.

If such arguments are true, how can we explain our faith in modern curative medicine? Has the rise of science banished magic only to replace it with a new religion, that of scientific biomedicine? Have we merely replaced one form of belief with another? One person who thinks so is the influential critic of modern medicine, the theologian Ivan Illich, whose article in the Course Reader (Part 3, Section 3.7) summarises many of the criticisms made against contemporary medicine. Turn to the Reader and, when you have read Illich's article, answer the following questions.

□ How has the pattern of disease changed over the last century in industrialised societies, according to Illich?

■ The traditional mass killers, the infectious diseases, have virtually disappeared. Most people now die of the diseases of old age.

□ What, does he argue, have been the main causes of this dramatic shift?

■ Better nutrition is the most important cause, but improvements in the wider environment, such as better housing and better work conditions, have also played major roles.

□ What part has ordinary medical practice played in creating this improved health?

■ Illich argues that its role has been crucial in some areas, for example, pernicious anaemia and polio, but its overall effect has been far less than the changes in the wider environment and in nutrition.

□ What part has ordinary medical practice had in actually creating new types of disease?

■ A major one, according to Illich. He lists as harmful the 'side-effects' of many new drugs and the consequences of what is often called 'unnecessary surgery'. For him, surgery and chemotherapy (drug treatment) are new forms of epidemic.

□ What other harmful effects, on this version, has the rise of this form of scientific medicine had?

■ It has made all of us its patients. We are now subordinate to medicine; medicine is becoming our master, not our servant. Our very humanity is at stake.

So popular faith in biomedicine has been seriously misplaced, at least according to Illich. Now that the more fatal epidemics are safely out of the way, modern medicine is creating its own, or so he argues. We shall now examine this charge by considering the history of plague (Chapters 4–6), hysterectomy (Chapter 7) and hysteria (Chapters 8 and 9): in turn, an epidemic of infectious disease — the greatest in our history; a possible surgical epidemic; and a possible diagnostic epidemic.

Objectives for Chapter 3

When you have studied this chapter, you should be able to:

3.1 Discuss some ways in which the various meanings of health are common to a great many different cultures.

3.2 Discuss the rights and duties involved in the sick role and the reasons for these.

3.3 Discuss the variety of healers available to patients in industrialised and more traditional societies.

3.4 Discuss the extent to which supernatural theories of disease-causation dominate traditional cultures, and the debate over this.

3.5 Discuss the way in which traditional medical theories have lingered on in twentieth-century popular beliefs.

3.6 Discuss the reasons for thinking that popular faith in biomedical science may be somewhat misplaced.

Questions for Chapter 3

1 (*Objective 3.2*) At the height of Stalin's drive to industrialise the Soviet Union faster than any country had previously managed, doctors were not allowed to give sickness certificates to more than a limited number of factory workers.

(a) What happened to the sick role in these circumstances?

(b) What does this suggest about the relationship between the sick role and society?

2 (*Objective 3.3*) Scientific medicine is only one of many types of medical tradition. List some examples of other traditions whose healers also practise in modern Western society.

3 (*Objective 3.6*) What are the main similarities and differences between the therapeutic nihilism of the nineteenth century, described in Chapter 2, and the modern therapeutic nihilism of Ivan Illich?

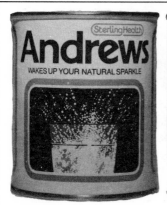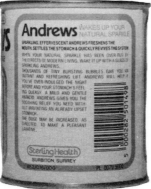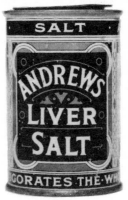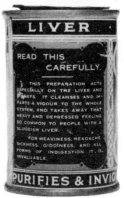

Figure 3.1 A modern tin of Andrews salts (*left*); and a 1911 tin of Andrews salts (*right*).

4 (*Objective 3.1*) The tin of 'Andrews salts' shown on the left in Figure 3.1 gives the following advice: 'When your natural sparkle has been over-run by the effects of modern living, wake it up with a glass of sparkling Andrews.'

This message refers directly to a theory of health that is found in all cultures, according to Dubos. What is it?

5 (*Objective 3.4*) '[Jesus] met ... a man with an unclean spirit who ... always night and day, ... was in the mountains, and in the tombs, crying and cutting himself with stones .... And Jesus asked him, 'What is thy name?' And he answered, saying, 'My name is Legion: for we are many.' ... Now there was nigh unto the mountains a great herd of swine feeding. And all the devils besought him saying, 'Send us into the swine, that we may enter them.' And forthwith Jesus gave them leave and the unclean spirits went out and entered into the swine: and the herd ran violently down a steep place into the sea ... and they were choked .... And [the people in the city] came to Jesus and saw him that was possessed with the devil and had the legion, sitting and clothed and in his right mind: and they were afraid.' (Mark 5: 2–15)

(a) What would we call a man with an unclean spirit today?

(b) What is unusual in modern Western terms about the cause of this man's condition, the way he is treated and the relation of Jesus to the cause?

(c) Are there any parallels between this description and those in contemporary societies?

6 (*Objective 3.5*) The 'Andrews' tin on the right in Figure 3.1 dates from 1911; its message has direct links to classical and medieval medical theory. One is the emphasis on the importance of the liver which, in that theory, secreted two of the four humours — yellow and black bile.

This preparation acts especially on the liver and kidneys. It cleanses and imparts a vigour to the whole system, and takes away that heavy and depressed feeling so common to people with a sluggish liver.

For heaviness, headache, sickness, giddiness, and all forms of indigestion it is invaluable.

Can you spot another reference to humoral theory?

4
Infectious disease and human history

In 1658, Oliver Cromwell died unexpectedly from 'ague' at the relatively early age of 59. His determination, organisational brilliance and military skill had been largely responsible, so many thought, for the Parliamentary victory in the English Civil War, and he had grown to dominate English political life. However, though there had been no serious challengers to his authority, upon his death the Stuart Kings were restored to the throne, when no stable republican alternative could be found. Had he lived another ten years, the course not only of English but of European history might have been quite different. Infectious disease — in this case almost certainly malaria — had claimed another victim.

The death of an individual may occasionally have repercussions across a whole society. Far more important, however, is the impact of infectious disease on entire populations of human beings. Indeed, there are some grounds for thinking that such disease has played a major role in the shaping of human history. It has shaped us, and we in our turn have shaped it. Exploring this will enable us to examine some of the complex relationships between the biological realm and the human social world.

The impact of infectious disease

One of the most important dates in human history is 1492. In that year, Christopher Columbus, an Italian sailor hired by the Queen of Spain, landed in the Americas and triggered an explosion of European expansion and conquest. The Spanish, and after them many other European nations, poured across the Atlantic, and it is mostly their descendants who inhabit and rule this huge continent. How did it come about that a handful of adventurers could colonise this vast territory? Traditionally, the European victory over the local Indian population was ascribed to the skill and the courage of the invaders, to the technologically primitive nature of American Indian

civilisation and to the relatively small number of Indians who lived there. None of these reasons now seems adequate. Archaeological and historical evidence reveals that civilisations such as those of the Incas and the Aztecs had sophisticated bureaucratic, military and architectural skills. They were, moreover, of enormous size. Whereas scholarly opinion used to put the total population of the continent at somewhere between 8 and 14 million people at the time that Columbus arrived, modern calculations suggest an overall population of around 100 million. Of these, 15 to 30 million were part of the Mexican civilisation and a similar number belonged to that of the Andes.

Yet by 1568, it is now estimated, the Indian population of central Mexico had shrunk from around 30 million to nearer 3 million, and was to fall even further, reaching a low of around 1.6 million in 1620. Throughout the Americas, the story was the same: a 90 per cent drop in population over a period of around 120 years. Little wonder, then, that it is mostly the descendants of the Europeans who now inhabit the Americas.

What can explain this extraordinary drop in population, and with it the complete destruction of the great Indian civilisations? The answer would seem to be the devastating impact of infectious diseases brought to the New World by the European invaders. The conquests of Cortez and Pizzaro in the 1520s were made possible by smallpox and the consequent total disruption of the Aztec and Inca empires. Yet more disease was to come. The 1530s saw an appalling outbreak of measles, also new to the Americas, whose first impact was as crippling as that of smallpox in the previous decade. In 1546 there came a wave of the typhus which had reached Europe a few years earlier. Likewise, a terrible 'flu epidemic, which had hit Europe in 1556, reached the Americas in 1558–59. Finally, in the seventeenth century, the importation of black slaves from Africa to replace the devastated local population brought with it two African diseases that found a ready home in the tropical rain forests of the central part of the continent: malaria and yellow fever. As one Indian chronicler recalled:

> Great was the stench of death. After our fathers and grandfathers succumbed half the people fled to the fields. The dogs and vultures devoured their bodies. The mortality was terrible. Your grandfathers died and with them the son of the King and his brothers and kinsmen. So it was that we became orphans, oh my sons. So we became when we were young. All of us were thus. We were born to die. (*The Annals of the Cakchiquels and Title of the Lords of Totonicapan*, quoted in McNeill, 1979, p.200)

The destruction of Amerindian civilisation is the most dramatic instance of the impact of infectious disease on human history. Other examples are more contentious or more complex. Nevertheless, some historians believe that a terrible epidemic which hit Greece in 430–429 BC gave Athens a blow from which it never recovered, and that the fall of the Roman Empire may have been due in part to the huge devastation caused by the great epidemics of AD 165–180, 251–266, 355–363 and 540–644.

Since the evidence is sparse, such ideas are likely to remain matters for conjecture. There is, however, much stronger evidence concerning the social impact of a more recent epidemic, the wave of cholera which swept across Europe in 1831–32. Cholera was far less devastating than the plagues which had hit American or Roman civilisation. It was nevertheless formidable. Glasgow, one of the worst affected places, suffered 3 000 deaths, and, in one week in August 1831, 228 Glaswegians died of the disease. The longer-term effect of the epidemic was to prove equally important. From the 1820s onwards, there had been a major political campaign in all Western nations for the reform of public health measures: for the clearance of slums, the provision of clean water and the construction of sewers — the movement for sanitary reform, as it was known. Cholera provided just the evidence for which the reformers had been searching; devastating though it was, its impact was partial — only the poorest really suffered, the rich mostly escaped (see Figure 4.1). Not everyone accepted this connection between bad living conditions and cholera but the nineteenth-century public health movement, which shaped the construction of all modern towns and cities, certainly owed something to the savage lesson taught in 1831.

Finally, note that although cholera, 'flu, bubonic plague, smallpox and measles have all, at times, swept across human societies with devastating effect, it must also be remembered that other, more insidious, infections may be continually present in a population, with slower but potentially no less damaging effects. Tuberculosis, malaria,

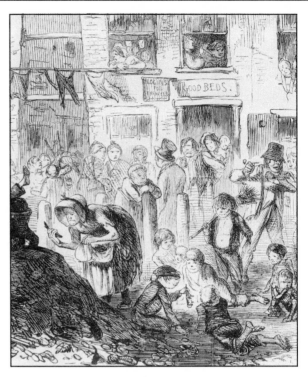

Figure 4.1 A court for King Cholera. (*Punch*, 1852)

the debilitating bilharzia or schistosomiasis (caused by flatworms) and sleeping sickness (carried by the tsetse fly) still place major limits on human life and human endeavour.

The human species and microorganisms

We have seen how infectious disease can lay rulers low and cause mighty empires to crumble into dust. Its particular impact on this or that civilisation may be disputed, but overall there seems little doubt of its power to shape human history. There are, however, some unanswered questions. For example, if measles and smallpox had such devastating effects on the American Indians, how did the Spanish conquerors who brought these infections with them remain *immune*? How is it that the same disease can cause one empire to collapse and another to replace it? The answer to this question lies in the complex relationship between human beings, the *microorganisms* that cause disease, the many other species which fill the planet, and the extraordinarily varied environments which they and we inhabit — environments which in turn are shaped by a multitude of climatic, geographical and social factors. An introduction to the topic can be gained from the work of the American historian William McNeill, who comments thus on the relationship of human beings, both to one another and to other species:

Disease and parasitism play a pervasive role in all life. A successful search for food on the part of one organism becomes for its host a nasty infection or disease. All animals depend on other living things for food, and human beings are no exception. Problems of finding food and the changing ways human communities have done so are familiar enough in economic histories. The problems of avoiding becoming food for some other organisms are less familiar, largely because from very early times human beings ceased to have much to fear from large-bodied animal predators like lions or wolves. Nevertheless, one can properly think of most human lives as caught in a precarious equilibrium between the micro-parasitism of disease organisms and the macro-parasitism of large-bodied predators, chief among which have been other human beings.
(McNeill, 1979, p.13)

Such a picture initially conjures up an image of mutually hostile species continually at war with one another. The full story is, however, rather different.

☐ What would happen, if each species preyed unrelentingly on another in its search for food?
■ A successful predator would rapidly use up its food supply.

In consequence, although microorganisms which live in human bodies find a valuable source of food or shelter in human tissues, those that provoke acute disease are in danger of destroying themselves also. Over time, therefore, there is a tendency for *mutual accommodation between species* to be reached*. Smallpox and measles, the diseases that devastated the Amerindians, are both classic examples of this tendency. Although their initial impact on human societies that have never experienced them before is

* This process of 'co-evolution' is discussed in more detail in *The Biology of Health and Disease*. The Open University (1985) *The Biology of Health and Disease*, The Open University Press. (U205 *Health and Disease*, Book IV)

catastrophic, those humans that survive have a degree of resistance, or natural immunity. After a few generations, measles and smallpox can still survive in such societies, but normally only as childhood diseases; occasionally lethal, but without the overwhelmingly destructive nature of their first arrival.

This process of mutual accommodation is the normal relationship between the human species and microorganisms, most forms of which live happily in the human gut or mouth, or on the skin, without causing any great disturbance. As we have seen, however, the relationship does sometimes have its problems; problems that we call disease.

☐ What might cause problems in the relationship?
■ One key factor has already been touched on — where the microorganism and a particular human population are new to each other, there has not yet been time for a process of accommodation to occur — if this is necessary. You might also have thought of the following: mutation in either the microorganism itself or in the human population; shifts in the wider environment of both species brought about by climatic, social or geological change; finally, whereas some microorganisms have only one host during their life cycle (for example, the virus that causes measles) and therefore have a relatively simple form of adaptation, others (such as the microorganisms involved in malaria and plague) have other hosts too such as mosquitos and fleas, as well as the human species, which exist in a complex relationship with one another.

The biological and social worlds are continuously *evolving*; a situation which may sometimes leave one species with a huge advantage over others. As we have seen, such an advantage often proves no more than temporary. Over time, each side may develop a degree of natural immunity to the impact of the other. The multicellular organism that causes malaria gradually becomes resistant to DDT; the human being develops some immunity to the worst ravages of the virus that causes measles.

Objective for Chapter 4

When you have studied this chapter, you should be able to:

4.1 Describe the relations between infectious disease and the human species, the process of accommodation that usually occurs, and the conditions under which such disease can have a major impact on human social life.

Question for Chapter 4

1 (*Objective 4.1*) Why did the measles and smallpox brought to America by the Spanish invaders devastate the Indians but spare the Spanish?

5

Plague: the three pandemics

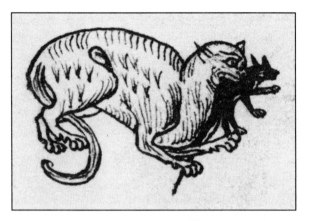

Figure 5.1 Cat with rat.

In Chapter 4 we described the impact of infectious disease on the development of human society. According to William McNeill, it not only devastated the Incas and the Aztecs but also helped to lay the Greek and Roman Empires low. And, according to the German historian, E. Friedell, one particular infection, bubonic plague, both destroyed traditional European society and in so doing created the conditions for the new Europe — the Europe that captured the Americas, the Europe of the Reformation and the Renaissance, of capitalism, science, democracy and global empire. These are big claims and heavily disputed by many writers. Just what is the evidence for them? How can we know precisely how many people died of smallpox in some epidemic in the remote past? How do we know that it was this, rather than some other disease, that was to blame? And, even if we know both these things, how can we assess the impact of epidemic disease on a society when there are so many other powerful forces, such as war, trade and famine, which also shape its destiny?

In this and the next chapter we shall try to answer some of these questions by focusing on the impact of a single disease, plague, on just one area of the world. We shall summarise some of the contemporary biomedical knowledge about plague and then attempt to apply this to surviving historical accounts. In doing so, we shall trace the course of plague in Europe over nearly 2000 years. The story culminates in the late nineteenth century with the scientific breakthroughs that have effectively lifted the enormous threat that plague posed for so long, at least for the time being.

Since plague has been the most devastating of all infectious diseases in the history of Europe, its historical trajectory has been studied more intensively than that of any other infectious disease. It therefore allows us to examine some of the complex interactions between the biological realm and the human social world. Having said this, note also that, despite intensive research going back well over a century, there is still much in the story that is controversial. As we shall see, there are doubts as well as certainties.

Plague: a biomedical review

Let us begin by examining what is currently known about plague on the biomedical side. Until the late nineteenth century, the word 'plague' (derived from a Latin word meaning a blow) was used to describe epidemics of many different diseases. However, following the work of two scientists in 1894, the Japanese, Shibasburo Kitasato (1852–1931), and the Frenchman, Alexander Yersin (1863–1943), the term is now applied specifically to the acute infectious disease caused by a microorganism, the bacillus *Yersinia pestis* (formerly called *Pasteurella pestis*).

There are, however, several complications to the biological story which we need to grasp if we are to understand the historical controversies in the rest of this chapter. (The key points to remember will be summarised at the end of this section.) First, the microorganism comes in several different forms, some deadly, others less so. Three major strains or varieties have been identified: *Yersinia pestis orientalis*, *Yersinia pestis antiqua* and *Yersinia pestis medievalis*. There are also several minor strains of plague which, though unpleasant enough as diseases, are considerably less deadly. Exposure to these minor forms immunises the sufferer against the major forms, just as cowpox immunises against smallpox.

Second, *Yersinia pestis* can affect the human body in three different ways. The most common form, known as *bubonic plague*, is characterised by the swellings which commonly develop, first as a blister or carbuncle at the site of the infection and later as 'buboes' (inflammatory swelling of the glands) in the groin, neck or armpits. If untreated, as all cases effectively were until the development of modern antibiotics in the 1940s, 60 per cent of all sufferers die, most of them within five days. The second form is a more severe version of the first called *septicaemic plague*, whose sufferers die even more quickly, normally within twenty-four hours and before there is time to develop buboes. A few, however, live just a little longer and develop a lung infection also. The coughing that this generates can occasionally pass the disease on to others, thus creating a third form of the illness, *pneumonic plague*. Here the infection is localised in the lungs and causes coughing, sneezing, bleeding from the nose and the spitting of blood. This third form of the disease is particularly virulent, killing 90 per cent of its victims, normally within three days of their being infected.

Third, although so far we have used the term epidemic to describe an outbreak of infectious disease, this is not the only important term to learn in this area. Where the microorganism that causes the disease has settled down in its host community, outbreaks of acute illness still occur, but they tend to be small and frequent. When this is so, the disease is held to be *endemic* within the community.

□ What infectious diseases are currently endemic within the UK?

■ A great many. You may have thought of measles, mumps, chicken pox, german measles, or others.

As we noted in Chapter 4, there is normally an accommodation over time between the microorganism that causes the disease and its host. Diseases that become endemic therefore tend to take a rather milder form after their first impact; indeed, many become 'childhood diseases' which most people experience early in life but from which most quickly recover. However, when, for whatever reason, the normal equilibrium is upset, or when the microorganism encounters a community which has no previous experience of the disease, it may spread with extraordinary rapidity throughout its host population. It is this which technically is known as an *epidemic*. (Epidemics which go on for a long time and spread very widely are known as *pandemics*.)

Now consider a fourth complexity, namely the number and variety of *hosts* off which the infectious microorganism lives. Some microorganisms, such as the virus which causes smallpox, have only one host — the human species — but others, such as *Yersinia pestis*, inhabit many different sorts of hosts, sometimes affecting one more than another and occasionally breaking out into a new source of food and shelter with startling rapidity and sometimes devastating effects.

Yersinia pestis is normally endemic within various types of wild rodent, a group of mammals which includes rats, mice, squirrels, beavers and guinea-pigs. Indeed, at least 220 different sorts of rodent have been discovered to be infected with *Yersinia*, and different rodents may harbour different strains (Christie, 1983). ('Enzootic' rather than endemic is the technical term for such infections among species other than ourselves, but we shall stick with endemic to make things simpler.) Of these various rodents, the rat is the most famous, but is far from the only sufferer.

In communities of ground-burrowing rodents, some relatively stable accommodation has been reached with the bacillus. *Yersinia pestis* is normally no more than a passing 'childhood' disease for these rodents and circulates in the population indefinitely, i.e. it is *endemic*. It is only when the disease invades previously unaffected rodent and human populations that extraordinary consequences can ensue.

Not only does *Yersinia pestis* infect rodents, it also infects the fleas that live in the rodents' fur and feed off the rodents' blood, thus passing the infection from one animal to another. The fleas' role is also important in transmitting the infection between rodents and human beings. There are some 2 000–3 000 types of flea, of which at least 30 are known to transmit plague. For plague to become epidemic, the right fleas and the right rodents must come together, their breeding seasons must be related and there must be plenty of active adult fleas around at the peak of the rodent breeding season. The temperature and humidity at which fleas are most active (15–20 °C and 90–95 per cent humidity) are therefore crucial factors in the *transmission* of the bubonic and septicaemic forms of plague. If it is too hot, too cold, or too dry, infected fleas are less likely to pass on the disease; indeed, at cold temperatures, a flea's own natural defence system is likely to destroy the harmful bacillus.

How then does the disease reach human beings? Fleas transfer from various rodents living in the wild to an intermediate host (another rodent, the rat) and from there they pass on to human beings. Rats are intermediate hosts because they live so close to human beings. *Rattus rattus*, the black rat, lives very close indeed, in houses, out-buildings or work-places, and is rarely found in fields. *Rattus norvegicus*, the brown rat, keeps at a slightly greater distance from human beings, living in sewers and in contact both with the black rat and with wild rodents. Both types of rat can develop some immunity to plague, particularly the brown rat, but neither seems to achieve the degree of accommodation that is found in some wild rodents.

The flea which transmits *Yersinia pestis* across these various other hosts is itself infected (though in a different manner from human beings) and eventually dies of dehydration, though not before providing ideal conditions for the reproduction and transmission of the microorganism. The passage from a flea's mouth to its stomach, known as the proventriculus, has seven rows of spines, and when the flea sucks blood, these interlock, then open rhythmically. This means that the blood first distends the proventriculus, then passes through to the stomach. If the flea bites an animal already infected with *Yersinia pestis*, the bacteria in the blood can quickly multiply, forming sticky colonies on the spines and gluing them together so that they can no longer open — a process known as 'blocking' (Figure 5.2). Now the flea sucks more avidly than ever, for no fluid can get through to its stomach. The blood meanwhile circulates around the proventriculus and is injected into the next animal the flea bites, taking *Yersinia pestis* with it. Soon the blocked and dehydrated flea dies, but by that time the disease has already been passed on to a new host.

□   What is the other means by which *Yersinia pestis* is transmitted?
■   The pneumonic form of the disease is passed directly in droplets of mucus from person to person by coughs and sneezes.

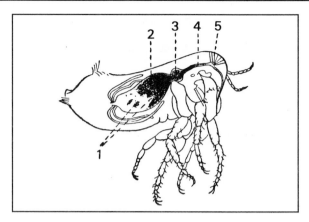

Figure 5.2 A 'blocked rat flea'. 1 Masses of *Yersinia pestis*. 2 Stomach. 3 Proventricular valve blocked with bacillary growth. 4 Oesophagus containing masses of *Yersinia pestis*. 5 Pharyngeal pump.

□   Which forms of the disease are likely to occur in the winter in Europe, which in the summer, and why?
■   Since pneumonic plague is passed directly from person to person, it can spread in either winter or summer. But the bubonic and septicaemic forms are more likely to be found in the summer since they are transmitted by fleas. Cold weather makes the fleas less active and also improves their natural defences against the disease.

The complex relationship between *Yersinia pestis* and its various hosts — rodents, fleas and human beings — explains both the devastating effects of plague when it initially breaks out and the complicated cycles of endemic and epidemic plague that seem to occur. In a human population which has never experienced bubonic plague or which has been free of it for many years, roughly 60 per cent of that population seem to become infected, and of these roughly 60 per cent die if they are untreated. In all, therefore, somewhere around 36 per cent of the total population die from the plague, a figure which is very similar to the estimates of the medieval chroniclers which we shall examine in a moment. Even higher rates of mortality occur when the plague also takes a pneumonic form.

What happens after this initial devastating outburst? As we shall see in the historical discussion that follows, the mortality during epidemics among human populations exposed to disease for many years does tend to be lower than that among newly exposed populations. One important reason for this is that pneumonic forms of plague seem less stable than the bubonic form and less likely to become endemic in a rodent population, so that pneumonic plague with its high mortality becomes less common in 'old' plague areas. In Europe during the sixteenth and seventeenth centuries, 15–20 per cent became an accustomed mortality in epidemics. The mortality in the Great Plague of London in 1665 was probably 17–18 per cent, and William Petty, the demographer and economist, said, 'In pestilential years (which are one in twenty) there dye of the people 1/6 of the plague and 1/5 of all diseases.' (Petty, 1667, p.18) That this was not the outcome of some developed human immunity is indicated by the continued occasional occurrence of some more severe epidemics: the mortality at Eyam in Derbyshire in 1665–66, for instance, was a little under 50 per cent, and at Marseille in 1720 the mortality was more than 50 per cent, according to the leading French plague historian, J. N. Biraben (1975).

Nevertheless, the overall mortality level does seem to decline after a while, apart from the occasional spectacular outburst. The one in Marseille, in fact, signalled the end of that particular wave of plague in Europe. What can account for all this? In Europe, neither rats nor people ever became fully accommodated to the disease; it never declined here into a childhood disease. Nevertheless, human populations which have experienced plague epidemics do develop some temporary resistance. Some people are naturally immunised in the process of recovery, and they act as buffers to the spread of infection throughout the population over periods of twenty or more years. This resistance, however, cannot be inherited and, as a new generation of non-immune children grows to form a significant proportion of the community, the whole population becomes increasingly vulnerable.

The same process also happens among the rat population. Rats seem to be able to transmit immunity to their offspring at least over two or three generations. But, as they breed faster than human beings, this immunity disappears more quickly than in human populations. There is thus an approximate five-year cycle of disease among rats from epidemic to epidemic. It was probably the somewhat irregular coincidence of twenty-year human cycles of generations and five-year rat cycles which was responsible for the long series of epidemics in Britain and Europe during the fifteenth, sixteenth and early seventeenth centuries.

The development of immunity among rats may also explain the fact that long periods of endemic plague among humans have often ended, not in a process of slow decline in the disease's incidence, but in a final severe epidemic, which some historians have called a 'fireball' effect. On this argument, a really severe epidemic is precipitated by environmental conditions favourable to fleas, and destroys all the non-immune rats that are left. The 'fireball' consumes everything vulnerable in its path before finally burning itself out.

Studying plague in history

Now that we have gained some idea of the basic biological aspects of *Yersinia pestis*, let us try to apply this to the historical understanding of the various forms of this plague that have swept Europe during the last 2 000 years. Let us begin, therefore, by recapping the key points that we have just covered: first, the bacillus occurs in several different strains; second, the process of the disease within the body can take a bubonic, septicaemic or pneumonic form; third, the bacillus has several hosts — various rodents, rats and fleas as well as human beings; fourth, it can be transmitted to human beings either indirectly via fleas or directly as in the pneumonic form, the latter enabling it to be spread during the winter as well as the summer months; and fifth, given its complex association with a range of different hosts, some of whom only develop partial immunity to its ravages, the disease occurs in a great variety of endemic and epidemic forms, breaking out here, dying down there, killing massively at one point, sparing most at another.

There are also a few complexities on the historical side. Again, there is no need to worry about all the details, but the following few points are worth bearing in mind. First, if all or most forms of epidemic were known in the past as 'plagues', how are we going to distinguish those caused by *Yersinia pestis* from all the other 'plagues' of history, from measles, smallpox, typhus and so on? In 1971, for example, the bacteriologist J.F. Shrewsbury tried to minimise the significance of plague, seeking to show, among other things, that much of the mortality attributed to plague was in fact the result of typhus, smallpox or other diseases. Yet another bacteriologist has recently claimed that it was anthrax, not plague, that was actually responsible for the Black Death of the fourteenth century. Determining whether a particular plague was in fact caused by *Yersinia pestis* will involve us in some detailed historical medical detective work.

Second, even if we do decide that a particular outbreak was indeed plague, we must bear in mind that much of our knowledge of plague is in fact based on historically recent epidemics in Asia of just one strain of the disease, *Yersinia pestis orientalis*. We cannot be absolutely sure that the 'ancient' and 'medieval' strains had exactly the same effects; indeed, historians disagree as to whether *antiqua* or *medievalis* was responsible for the great epidemic of the fourteenth century. More generally, there is always a problem in extrapolating from contemporary knowledge to the past. Third, how should we assess the impact of plague when there were so many other factors such as periodic crop failures and starvation which might be as, or more important, a cause of mortality?

Fourth, just how *reliable* are the medieval records and chronicles? Records survive from only a few places and may not be typical of other areas. And, given the general devastation caused by plague, just how accurate are the chroniclers' observations? May they not have exaggerated its effects? As we shall see, there are many vivid accounts of the impact of the Black Death in Britain, in chronicles, official documents and estate records. But the limitations of this historical source material has allowed scholars to develop widely differing points of view. For example, radically different estimates of population size and plague mortality have been suggested. In the absence of census records, of what value, it is asked, are contemporary estimates like the 100 000 deaths in Venice and the 50 000 in Paris, or John of Fordun's assessment of a one-third mortality in Scotland?

Finally, in addition to the problems of identifying plague, the uncertainty over the precise strain involved, the possible unreliability of medieval observers and the absence of certain forms of systematic record, there is a problem of terminology. The rest of this chapter contains a detailed historical reconstruction of the course of the three great European pandemics. The word 'pandemic' was adopted by medical historians during the nineteenth century to describe lengthy and widespread epidemics. It has been used in the study of plague to identify three such prolonged epidemics which have affected the European world in recorded history. However, though many recent textbooks still use the term, William McNeill criticises its use and points out that it has misleading implications. The most obvious is that it embodies a western European view of plague history. Plague has almost certainly been endemic among rodents in large parts of Africa and Asia, including the eastern seaboards of the Mediterranean, throughout historic times. Only when plague has become epidemic and spilled over into the western European rodent population, thereby becoming endemic here, have European historians described the results as a 'pandemic'. However, as long as this reservation is kept in mind, the word 'pandemic' is a helpful one in the analysis of issues in plague history. It is useful, at least in a European context, to have a term which distinguishes between those periods in which plague was endemic in the rodent population and those in which it was not.

Using this term, many Western historians have identified a first pandemic which occurred in the European classical world and was recorded in Graeco-Roman literature, and ended around AD 650. There was then a gap until a second, and better recorded, pandemic that entered from the Near East in 1347–48 and manifested itself in periodic epidemics for nearly 400 years; in Britain its end is marked conventionally by the London plague of 1665 and in Europe by the Marseille plague of 1720–22. It was for the terrible early stages of this pandemic that the term 'Black Death' was invented many years later. The third, and most recent, pandemic, which in some senses we are still experiencing, is conventionally said to have begun in China in 1890: it reached India in 1894 and Britain in 1900. During this third pandemic, progress in the identification and treatment of the disease enabled various health authorities to control its spread and to prevent it taking a hold in many, though not all, of the major centres of population. All three pandemics will be described in what follows, but the second of these will be discussed at greater length since it dramatically illustrates the interrelationship of disease and social development in medieval and early modern societies. So let us now look at the evidence and see how far we can identify the causes, nature and course of the great European plagues.

The first pandemic

The date of the onset of the first European pandemic is difficult to establish. The Philistines (about 1100 BC) suffered the plague of the city of Ashdod, a plague associated with mice and with what the Authorised Version of the Bible translates as 'emerods' (haemorrhoids) but which seems quite possibly to have been the plague buboes: 'the hand of the Lord was against the city with a very great destruction: and he smote the men of the city, both small and great, and they had emerods in their secret parts' (I Samuel 5: 9). To propitiate the God of Israel, the Philistines are said to have given in offering five golden emerods and five golden mice.

☐　What suggests this might have been plague?
■　The fact that the 'emerods' occurred in the groin, as do buboes, and the mice — a form of rodent.

It is less certain that the famous plague of Athens (430–428 BC) was bubonic plague; some historians believe that it was typhus. But there is little doubt that the great epidemic of the reign of the Emperor Julian (AD 355–363), and described by his physician Oribasius, was bubonic plague: 'the buboes called pestilential are most fatal and acute ... [the illness was] accompanied by acute fever, pain and prostration of the whole body, delirium, and the appearance of large and hard buboes, which did not suppurate ... in the groins and armpits.' (quoted in Crawfurd, 1914, p.76)

The last great epidemic of ancient times first appeared at Antioch in Syria in AD 540, then crossed the continent from south-east to north-west, and ended, in AD 644, as a notorious outbreak in Ireland and Wales known as the plague of Cadwalader's time. This particular epidemic had been closely observed in Byzantium (Istanbul) in AD 542 by the historian Procopius:

... [the epidemic] seemed to move by fixed arrangement, and to tarry for a specific time in each

country ... [it] always took its start from the coast, and from there went up to the interior ... it reached Byzantium in the middle of spring, ... [victims] had a sudden fever, some when just roused from sleep, others while walking about, others while otherwise engaged, without any regard to what they were doing ... a bubonic swelling developed; and this took place not only in the particular part of the body which is called 'bubon' [groin], that is, below the abdomen, but also inside the armpit, and in some cases also beside the ears, and at different points on the thighs ... those who were seized with delirium suffered from insomnia and were victims of a distorted imagination; for they suspected that men were coming upon them to destroy them, and they would become excited and rush off in flight, crying out at the top of their voices ... death came in some cases immediately, in others after many days; and with some the body broke out with black pustules about as large as a lentil and these did not survive even one day, but all succumbed immediately. With many also a vomiting of blood ensued without visible cause and straightway brought death ... the disease in Byzantium ran a course of four months, and its greatest virulence lasted about three ... the tale of dead reached five thousand each day, and again it even came to ten thousand and still more than that.
(Procopius, 1914, pp.455–65)

☐   Which phrases suggest the occurrence in Byzantium of the bubonic, septicaemic and pneumonic forms of plague? (Look back at the first part of the chapter if necessary.)
■   Bubonic — 'a bubonic swelling developed'; septicaemic — 'these did not survive even one day'; pneumonic — 'with many also a vomiting of blood ensued without visible cause'.

It is detailed clinical descriptions such as those given by Procopius which suggest that these ancient epidemics were indeed plague, rather than typhus, anthrax or some other infectious disease. As we noted in Chapter 2, the detailed clinical description of disease was still in its infancy even in the days of Sydenham, and it is therefore often impossible to identify particular diseases from historical accounts. Plague, however, has several highly distinctive features which justify analysis of this kind.

After AD 644 plague disappeared from western Europe for 700 years. The circumstances in which this 'first pandemic' disappeared, during the period conventionally known as the Dark Ages, are, and are likely to remain, obscure.

The second pandemic in Europe

Traditional accounts link the immediate source of the second pandemic in western Europe to Tartar (Mongol) armies who were then active around the shores of the Black Sea. Asia Minor and the Black Sea coasts were at that time in regular trading contact with Venice, Genoa and other Italian ports. The arrival at Messina in Sicily from the Black Sea of a fleet of Genoese galleys containing plague victims in October 1347 probably marks the onset of the disease. Whether the disease was then in a primary pneumonic form among the crews or carried by fleas on shipborne rats is not known. During the following six months similar landings were made in most of the major ports of the western Mediterranean. Venice was one of the ports affected, and was among the first to attempt practical preventative measures. By March 1348 the arrival of ships was carefully controlled. The Venetian Republic was one of the wealthiest and best-administered states in Europe, and the forty-day quarantine that it later established for ships entering the port was adopted as a standard procedure by many other cities in Italy and elsewhere in Europe. ('Quarantine' comes from the Italian word for forty, 'quaranta', and also refers to Christ's forty days in the wilderness.) However, since no one knew how plague was transmitted until the beginning of this century, these and other measures proved incapable of preventing an extraordinarily severe epidemic in the city, and a consequent mortality estimated by contemporaries at 100 000.

☐   Why might quarantine fail to prevent the transmission of plague?
■   Strict quarantine might prevent the passage of the pneumonic form but, since the bubonic and septicaemic forms are transmitted by rat fleas, quarantine would work only if rats as well as people were unable to pass.

The plague reached Florence, another of the great cities of fourteenth-century Europe, a month after Venice. The classic Italian collection of short stories, *The Decameron*, written by the Florentine Boccaccio were supposedly told by members of the local nobility who had fled from the plague to a country house. In this book Boccaccio gave a graphic account of the arrival of the epidemic and of the attempted public health measures.

In the year of Our Lord 1348, there happened at Florence a most terrible plague; which whether owing to the influence of the planets, or that it was sent from God as a just punishment for our sins, had broken out some years before in the Levant, and after passing from place to place, and making incredible havoc all the way, had now reached the west. There, in spite of all the means that art and human foresight

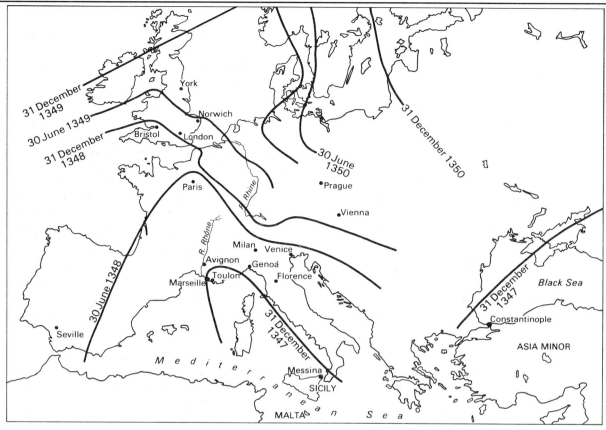

Figure 5.3 The spread of the Black Death in Europe, 1348–50.

could suggest, such as keeping the city clear from filth, the exclusion of all suspected persons, and the publication of copious instructions for the preservation of health, and notwithstanding manifold supplications offered to God in processions and otherwise; it began to show itself in the spring of the aforesaid year, in a sad and wonderful manner. Unlike what had been seen in the east, where bleeding from the nose is the fatal prognostic, here there appeared certain tumours in the groin or under the armpits, some as big as a small apple, others as an egg; and afterwards purple spots in most parts of the body; in some cases large and but few in number, in others smaller and more numerous — both sorts the usual messenger of death. To cure of this malady, neither medical knowledge nor the power of drugs was any effect ... (Boccaccio, 1855, pp.1–2)

In France, plague arrived in the port of Marseille in the autumn of 1347 but, perhaps because of cold weather, took several months to become established in the surrounding district. It reached Avignon, then the seat of the Pope, only in January 1348. The Pope's physician, Guy de Chauliac,

was another contemporary who observed the disease with great care:

> The disease was of two sorts: the first lasted two months (January and February), with continuous fever and expectoration of blood; and men died of it in three days. The second lasted the remainder of the time, also with continuous fever and with external carbuncles and buboes, chiefly in the armpit or the groin, and men died of it in five days. (quoted in Morris, 1977, p.39)

☐   What evidence do the quotations from Boccaccio and de Chauliac provide for the occurrence of pneumonic and bubonic plague in Florence and Avignon? Did the epidemics in the two cities differ?

■   The epidemics in the two cities were clearly different. Boccaccio saw only bubonic plague ('tumours under the groin') — though he knew about pneumonic plague ('bleeding from the nose'), he evidently did not observe it in Florence. De Chauliac observed both the pneumonic ('expectoration of blood') and the bubonic forms of plague in Avignon.

The epidemic spread northwards to Paris in May: one chronicler estimated that 50 000 people died there. In a number of places in France the surviving records are full enough for us to be able to calculate the mortality fairly accurately. The village of Givry in Burgundy, for instance, was one of the few in Europe for which parish registers from the fourteen century survive. These suggest that in 1340 the population was something over 1 200. In about three months in the summer of 1348, 615 people died, a mortality of 50 per cent. There is evidence of similar mortalities in both villages and towns in northern France.

The Black Death spread throughout western Europe between early 1348 and the summer of 1350 (see Figure 5.3). At first, it seemed to lose some of its virulence as it spread into the colder eastern regions and the less densely populated areas of central Europe. The Scandinavian countries, however, suffered severely in late 1349 and 1350, the colder weather seemingly having little effect on the course of the disease. We last hear of this great epidemic in the far north, in Iceland and in the Norse settlements in Greenland, which are thought to have been wiped out by the plague, leaving Greenland uninhabited and the Norse contacts with pre-Columbian America an almost forgotten legend.

☐ What could explain the way in which the plague was first seemingly checked by colder weather and then later broke out with great virulence in some of the coldest parts of Europe?
■ The bubonic and septicaemic forms are transmitted by fleas which are only active in warm weather. However, if a pneumonic form developed, this would not be checked by the cold.

After the Black Death, plague seems to have remained endemic in rats in western Europe for more than three centuries, bursting out occasionally in the human population much as the smallpox and measles endemic to the Spaniards had spread as epidemics among the Incas and Aztecs. As we shall see, however, the later human epidemics, though often severe, apparently became more localised in character. The Milan plague of 1630 was especially notorious, for there was an outbreak of savagery in which supposed plague spreaders were publicly tortured and burned alive.

There was then a brief lull in the occurrence of the disease but this was followed by a number of severe epidemics between the 1660s and the 1720s. The epidemic which so notoriously affected London in 1665–66 also affected the Rhineland, the Netherlands and France from 1666 to 1672. Then, after another brief lull, plague recurred again around the Mediterranean and in central Europe. There were widely reported epidemics in Malta, Vienna, Prague and throughout Germany from 1675 to 1683.

Finally, the second pandemic culminated in a major epidemic in Marseille, Toulon and Provence in 1720–22. The attention given to the Marseille epidemic was a measure both of its severity and the steady development of objective methods of observation and analysis among the doctors and public health authorities of the time. The elaborate costume worn by doctors to ward off plague in this period is shown in Figure 5.4.

After 1720–22 plague disappeared from western and central Europe for 150 years, apart from occasional port epidemics and isolated cases among travellers. The very severity of the epidemics in London, Marseille and elsewhere has been supposed in itself to have caused this disappearance.

☐ Why might a particularly severe epidemic bring a long period of plague to an end?
■ This is the so-called 'fireball' effect. There are two steps in this argument. First, over time, a degree of natural immunity builds up in the host populations. Second, if there are particularly favourable environmental conditions for the transmission of the microorganism, the epidemic quickly passes to all the non-immune members and burns itself out.

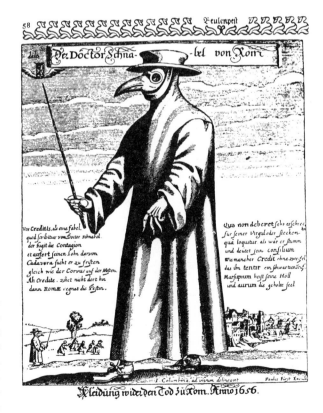

Figure 5.4 Protective clothing to ward off the plague.

The second pandemic in Britain

After this European survey of the second pandemic, let us turn to examine its course in Britain in more detail. A chronicle kept by Franciscan friars at King's Lynn in Norfolk, suggests that the Black Death first arrived in the country in June 1348 at Melcombe in Dorset, now called Weymouth. Another contemporary writer believed that Southampton, Bristol and London were also possible arrival points. However, what we know of the early stages of the epidemic is consistent with a June arrival in Dorset, followed by a slow spread into the rural hinterland during July and August, presumably associated with the development of endemic plague within the rat populations. Then, in the late summer, the disease advanced more rapidly, reaching larger centres of population — Southampton, Bristol, Gloucester and Exeter (Figure 5.5) — and at the same time taking on a more virulent form. The evidence from southern England has parallels with de Chauliac's observations from Avignon: once the particular bubonic strain in 1348 had established itself within the rat populations, a secondary and virulent pneumonic form appeared. In part of southern England, in fact, the epidemic gathered momentum during the winter of 1348–49.

The small town of Titchfield in Hampshire provides us with a dramatic example of the impact on one community. Titchfield stands at the head of a small estuary, ten miles east of Southampton, and plague may well have arrived there directly from France. At all events, the epidemic had broken out in the town by October 1348, the death of an unusual number of its abbey's tenants being reported in the manorial court held on 31 October. The high point of the epidemic was reached in the following March, and it ended in early May 1349. It was therefore a winter epidemic, almost certainly largely pneumonic in character. This seems to be confirmed by the very heavy mortality — 126 tenants were reported as dead, more than 60 per cent of all the tenants on the Titchfield estate. Most of the tenants were men of mature age. We have less evidence of the mortality among women, children, and landless men, but that this too was heavy is suggested by the fate of a hamlet

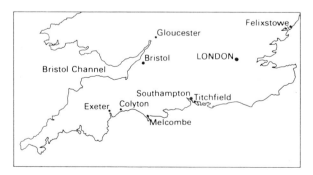

Figure 5.5 The coming of the Black Death to England and Wales.

called Quob in woodland north of the town. It was recorded in 1350 that: 'To this court came Thomas Schad for the tithingman [local official] of Quob and witnessed that all and each of the tithing died in the present pestilence ...'

The impact of the Black Death on this coastal district between Southampton and Portsmouth seems to have been particularly severe. On the abbey's estates, 305 out of 515 tenants died in 1348–49, a mortality a little under 60 per cent, and in 1361–62, in what was probably a bubonic epidemic, a further 92 died, a mortality of about 20 per cent among a reduced number of tenants. Plague was presumably now endemic among the local rodent population.

The Black Death reached London in September 1348, and moved up the east coast to Norwich in January 1349 and to York in May. It had already crossed the Bristol Channel into Wales by April 1349 and was there described by the Welsh poet Ieuan Gethin:

> Woe is me of the shilling in the armpit; it is seething, terrible, wherever it may come, a head that gives pain and causes a loud cry, a burden carried under the arms, a painful angry knob, a white lump. It is of the form of an apple, like the head of an onion, a small boil that spares no one. (quoted in Zeigler, 1970, p.197)

Later in the year the epidemic reached Ireland, and it is from Kilkenny that we have perhaps the most dramatic of all medieval accounts of the disease, written by Friar John Clyn during the epidemic itself:

> ... being myself as it were among the dead, waiting for death to visit me, [I] have put into writing truthfully all the things that I have heard. And, lest the writing should perish with the writer of the work and fail with the labourer, I leave parchments to continue this work, if perchance any may survive and any of the race of Adam escape this pestilence to carry on the work I have begun. (quoted in Morris, 1977, p.40)

At the end of this account Clyn wrote the words 'great hardship' and does, indeed, appear to have died; he is another of the contemporary observers who records the pneumonic symptom, the spitting of blood. The epidemic spread to Scotland somewhat later, in the spring of 1350, but lost none of its virulence in that time. The chronicler John of Fordun thought that a third of the population had died there.

Once firmly established in the local rat population, plague took on a rather different character. Centres, or *foci*, of the disease developed in many towns and throughout the countryside. Historians have listed a long series of epidemic years in Britain between 1348 and 1665, years in which plague, if not present throughout the country, can be detected in several provinces and a number of towns, often occurring in those cyclical patterns of fifteen or twenty years which are the results of temporary phases of immunity in the rodent and human populations. The American historian R.S. Gottfried has studied one particular area in great detail. He shows that, during the fifteenth century, plague was endemic in rural East Anglia, and that there were some eleven or twelve small groups of villages in which epidemics were both more frequent and more severe than elsewhere. He suggests that at that period epidemics developed in two different ways: by geographic spread along lines of communication and by 'spontaneous combustion' within endemic areas (perhaps in weather conditions particularly favourable to fleas).

In the sixteenth century, estimates of mortality began to be more precise. Major cities in Europe began to produce regular *Bills of Mortality*, listing all the people who had died recently and the causes of their deaths (see Figure 5.6). Such Bills are the origin of modern mortality statistics and were first produced to estimate the ravages of plague. On this basis, it seems that mortality in London during a severe epidemic in 1563 was between 18 and 25 per cent. The historian Paul Slack (1977) has calculated the mortality in

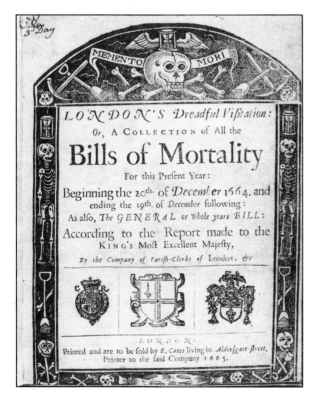

Figure 5.6 Title-page of the collected Bills of Mortality for London in the plague year, 1665.

Bristol in each of three epidemics in 1565, 1575 and 1603–4 as 16–18 per cent; and the Hampshire historian T.B. James (1983) gives a similar figure — 18 per cent — for an epidemic in Southampton in 1604.

Thus, although the death-rate was now halved, plague epidemics in the first two-thirds of the seventeenth century were still severe and of long duration. One episode from that period has been particularly carefully studied by the Cambridge demographer E.A. Wrigley and several others (Schofield, 1977). It took place in the Devon parish of Colyton in 1646. Colyton, a small town surrounded by hamlets, has many similarities to Titchfield in Hampshire, though here we can analyse the epidemic from the evidence of the parish registers rather than manorial rolls. Plague seems to have already been endemic in Colyton parish, but the main epidemic began in the first week of April, reached a high point in the first week of July, and was active until mid-October. This was, therefore, most likely an epidemic of bubonic plague. During those seven summer months some 330 of Colyton's population of 1 500 died, in comparison with an average of 67 from all causes in previous years; the deaths of some 260 people, or about 17 per cent of the population, can be attributed to plague. However, it is interesting to note that the deaths were confined to 48 per cent of the families in the parish; 52 per cent escaped unscathed.

☐ How might we account for the sharp division in Colyton between the 52 per cent of households completely free from plague and the unfortunate 48 per cent, in many of which more than one person died?

■ Some geographical factor which shaped the distribution of infected rats would seem the most obvious answer. For example, it seems plausible that the households of more remote farms might have escaped while those in the town suffered. (A similar 'patchiness' has been observed in modern epidemics in areas of endemic plague in Asia.) Unfortunately, the parish register does not tell us where the various families lived, so we cannot confirm the hypothesis for Colyton.

Colyton is, in fact, an example of the way in which areas of endemic plague in England slowly contracted during the seventeenth century. Just as within Colyton itself it seems possible that only part of the parish was affected, so in the surrounding countryside none of the seven adjacent parishes show any signs of plague in 1646. And this also proved to be the last epidemic in that part of Devon. There was still, however, the occasional violent outbreak elsewhere.

In the Great Plague of 1665 more than 68 000 deaths, almost certainly an underestimate, were recorded in London (see Figure 5.7). This was also the epidemic which reached the parish of Eyam in Derbyshire, where the Rector

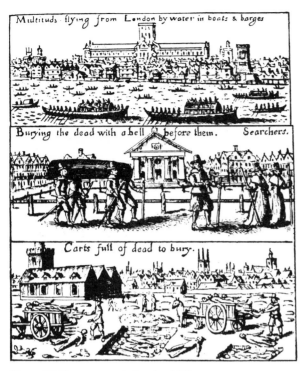

Multituds flying from London by water in boats & barges

Burying the dead with a bell before them. Searchers.

Carts full of dead to bury.

Figure 5.7 Plague scenes in London 1665.

organised a famous quarantine. All the inhabitants stayed inside the infected village to prevent the disease spreading, and food was left for them at a boundary stone. A total of 259 parishioners died. The event is vividly remembered in the locality, which still holds an annual service of remembrance. Overall, however, the English plague foci contracted yet again. Many northern and western counties seem to have escaped the last great epidemic of 1665–66, and in those counties which were affected the outbursts were confined to five or six foci. One of these was the small Hampshire town of Petersfield, about which the diarist Pepys recorded the interesting story that all the deaths occurred on one side of the street, the inhabitants on the other side remaining unscathed. After 1671 there is no record at all of plague in Britain for many years.

The third pandemic

After the Marseille and Toulon epidemics of 1720–22, plague ceased to affect Europe and the western Mediterranean regularly. Nevertheless, the disease remained endemic in parts of the Near East, periodically making an excursion westwards, to Messina in Sicily in 1743 and to Marseille in 1819. As such it remained a potential threat. When the European cholera epidemics began in 1831 anxious parallels were drawn between cholera and historic plague. In the next generation, therefore, European

observers journeyed deep into 'mysterious' Asiatic Russia to bring back new scientific evidence from what were seen as the heartlands of the disease. Just as they were doing so, a new plague epidemic was gathering force in northern China. It finally erupted into the ports used by European and American shipping companies in the 1890s, and in the process was characterised as a 'third pandemic'. The epidemic reached Hong Kong in 1890, Formosa in 1896 and San Francisco, Sydney and Glasgow in 1900. The most seriously affected country was India, then part of the British Empire. Hirst (1953) estimates that 13 100 000 people died as a result of this pandemic (1894–1938), of whom 12 500 000 were Indian (for comparison, 71 000 Japanese were killed by the immediate impact of the Hiroshima bombing).

It was in one sense fortunate, at least for Europe, that a third pandemic should have manifested itself in the 1890s. Louis Pasteur, pioneer of studies of microorganisms, had only recently retired from his research post at the Sorbonne; Robert Koch, who had identified the bacillus that causes tuberculosis, had just become Director of the new Institute of Infectious Disease in Berlin. Both men were popular heroes. On hearing reports of plague on the Chinese coast in 1894, the French and German governments promptly dispatched research teams. Results came rapidly. Pasteur's pupil, Alexander Yersin, and Koch's student, Shibasburo Kitasato, are usually credited with the identification of the plague bacillus. Yersin also drew attention to the probable role of rats, though he thought that the likely insect carriers were flies rather than fleas. It was 1898 before the French epidemiologist, P.L. Simond, pointed to the flea as the agent of transmission, and another decade before his thesis was widely accepted. Detailed studies of rats and wild rodent colonies were undertaken in the years that followed. A successful vaccine was developed in 1897, and a much improved version in 1938. However, in spite of rapid progress in the scientific understanding of the disease, and the introduction of much improved public health measures throughout the world, the plague of the 'third pandemic' established itself well beyond its previous foci. Indeed, once again, plague became endemic among the rat population of Britain, though its effects were far, far less than in previous outbreaks. There were sixteen deaths in a rapidly contained epidemic in Glasgow in 1900, and eight deaths in Liverpool in 1901.

The events along the estuary of the River Orwell near Felixstowe in Suffolk between 1908 and 1918 have been intensively studied and provide us with the most helpful evidence for the interpretation of the more extensive epidemics in the past. Plague appears to have reached this largely rural area by way of a rat or rats from a ship moored in the Thames Estuary. The disease spread widely through the rodent population; indeed, infected rats were found as far away as the suburbs of Ipswich. It was then transmitted, presumably by fleas, to the families living in several small groups of isolated cottages. At this point, a secondary pneumonic form developed that was responsible for most of the eighteen deaths that occurred in Suffolk.

The health authorities, after several weeks of confusion, finally acted vigorously. The principal control methods used were the destruction of refuse which might harbour rodents and the killing of the rodents themselves; some 250 000 rats were killed in Suffolk, as well as numbers of rabbits, ferrets and other animals. Only a small proportion of the rats examined were infected, which means that the disease had become endemic (present within the rodent population) rather than epidemic (sweeping rapidly through it). The last infected rats were identified in 1914, but human cases, apparently contracted in a pneumonic form, occurred until 1918. As a final control measure, a National Rat Week was declared in 1919 to try to stamp out the menace.

☐   Look back at the description of the arrival of plague in Dorset and Hampshire in 1348. What light do you think the Suffolk evidence from 1908–18 throws on the arrival of the Black Death at that time?

■   The spread of endemic plague in 1908–18, following what was probably a single contact with an infected ship, and then followed by the appearance of secondary pneumonic plague, looks very similar to the arrival of plague in Dorset and the appearance of pneumonic plague in Hampshire four months later. But we must not take such comparisons too far: the strain of plague in 1908, which had arrived in England from China, may have been different from the strain which arrived in 1348 from the Black Sea via Europe.

One strikingly new feature of the third pandemic also deserves comment: its much greater geographical spread. Unlike a number of other diseases, plague does not seem to have crossed the Atlantic into the Americas between the fifteenth and the nineteenth centuries. We can only suppose that the sea-crossing was then so slow that the disease had 'worked itself out' in humans, fleas and rats before landfall. Perhaps understandably, we have no first-hand accounts of such voyages, though the theme of an ill-fated plague ship, with the crew dead and the body of the skipper tied to the wheel, was a popular one in fiction. During the third pandemic, however, plague finally reached the Americas, presumably due to faster shipping. It has since remained endemic in the western states of the United States, in Mexico, Brazil, Argentina and elsewhere. Moreover, although it had probably been endemic in parts of equatorial Africa from the earliest times, during the third pandemic plague reached southern Africa by sea (see Figure 5.8) and spread right across North Africa; Albert Camus' novel, *The Plague*, is based on an actual epidemic in Oran in the 1940s.

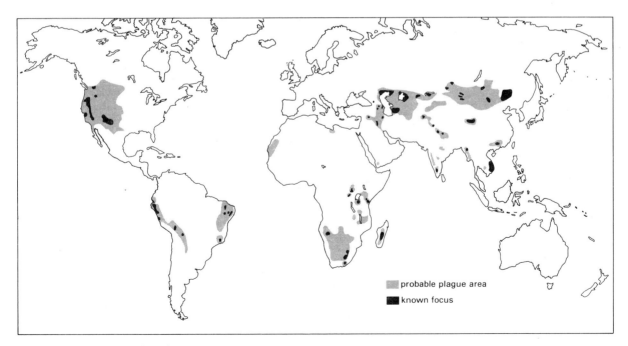

Figure 5.8 Contemporary plague foci.

Despite this greater geographical spread of plague and the appalling mortality in India in the early part of this century, the third pandemic has witnessed the first successful human attempts to combat its ravages. The vaccines, antibiotics and improved public health measures of modern medical science seem to have lifted its terrible threat. Nevertheless, since it is now endemic in many parts of the world, it still requires both constant vigilance and vigorous action by health authorities. Such measures may well have been helped by the development of insecticides. Their use for many other purposes seems to have had the incidental effect of reducing flea populations.

Thus, in recent years, there has been a steady decline in the number of cases reported to the World Health Organization: from over 4 400 cases and 100 deaths in 1970, to 172 cases and 17 deaths in 1982 — the smallest number since modern statistics have been collected. These last cases were, however, extremely widespread, being reported in Vietnam in Asia; in South Africa, Zimbabwe, Tanzania, Zaïre and Madagascar in Africa; and in Brazil, Peru, Bolivia and the United States in the Americas. In less developed countries plague is still normally associated with rat-infested villages and overcrowded suburbs; in more developed countries it more often occurs with the hunting and skinning of rodents. Vietnam is a special case. The origin of modern plagues here seems to lie in the disturbance of a previously stable relationship between humans and rodents by war and the attendant social disruption.

Objectives for Chapter 5

When you have studied this chapter, you should be able to:

5.1 Describe some of the problems in interpreting historical evidence concerning epidemic disease.

5.2 Describe the varieties of *Yersinia pestis*, its relationship to its various hosts, the various means by which it is transmitted from one to another and the eventual development of scientific understanding of the disease.

5.3 Describe the course of the three great European pandemics.

Questions for Chapter 5

1 (*Objective 5.1*) Because monks were literate, we have a disproportionate number of surviving accounts of the impact of the Black Death on monasteries. As an example, the chronicler of Meaux Abbey near Hull, writing at the beginning of the fifteenth century, reported that when the epidemic arrived there it killed the abbot and 6 monks on one day (12 August 1349), and a further 34 of the 50 monks and lay brothers in succeeding weeks, a mortality of 80 per cent. How reliable do you think this is as historical evidence?

2 (*Objective 5.2*) McNeill describes the arrival of plague in the Americas during the third pandemic in the following fashion:

... infected ship's rats and their fleas not only conveyed plague bacilli to human hosts ... but also managed to infect their wild cousins in several semi-arid regions of the earth. Apparently in California, Argentina and South Africa, potential wild reservoirs for bubonic infection had existed for incalculable ages. All that was needed to create new natural plague foci was a means to convey the bacillus across intervening barriers (in this case oceans) to new regions where suitably massive populations of burrowing rodents were already in the ground. Such rodent populations proved both susceptible to the disease and capable of sustaining an unbroken chain of infection indefinitely, despite wide local differences of habitat and speciation. (McNeill, 1979, p.148)

(a) What are the special roles of the rat, the flea, the human being and the wild rodent in the transmission of plague?

(b) What is the technical term used to describe the relationship between an infectious disease and a host population when that population is both 'susceptible to the disease and capable of sustaining an unbroken chain of infection indefinitely'?

(c) Since plague was new to the Americas, why did it become established only among the rodent population and not the human population?

3 (*Objective 5.2*) The people of Eyam were heroic. Rather than flee the plague, they kept themselves completely isolated while the plague raged among them; 259 of them died. Was their sacrifice of any use?

4 (*Objective 5.3*) Look at Figure 5.3 and at the description of the spread of the Black Death in Europe. The plague epidemic had severe effects in Scandinavia, but petered out as it spread eastwards into central Europe. Can you suggest explanations for these differences?

6

Plague: biological and social dimensions

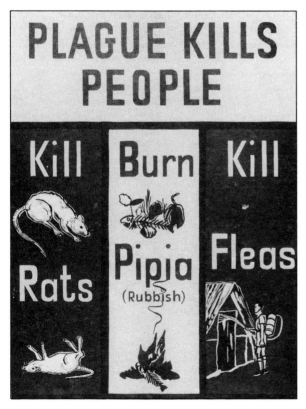

Figure 6.1 A modern Papua New Guinea plague poster.

By the late nineteenth century, the threat of plague, a threat that had hung over Europe for nearly 2000 years had begun to lift. But it would be wrong to end the story there. Several important questions about plague still need an answer. Where does it come from? Why did it sweep across Europe, stay for several centuries and then leave — and this at least twice in Europe's history? How did people try to explain the complex patterns and multitude of forms in which plague appeared before the discoveries of Kitasato, Yersin and Simond? Finally, since infectious disease (along with the Spaniards) seems to have destroyed the Aztec and Inca empires, what were the social and economic effects of plague in Europe? Was there similar destruction here?

In this chapter we consider some of these questions. Doing so raises once more the wider issue with which we began this study of infectious disease: that of the relationship between change in the biological realm and change in the human social world. We therefore end this case study with some further reflections on the place of human beings in the natural world and the kinds of factors which shape their lives and health. For the moment, however, let us think further about plague.

More medical detective work

Where did plague originally come from? Nowadays, *Yersinia pestis* is to be found in all regions of the world where there are large underground 'cities' of burrowing rodents. But most of these foci of infection are very recent. Three centres do, however, seem a good deal older: one in central Asia, somewhere between Tibet, Mongolia and Lake Baikal; one scattered across the length of the Eurasian steppe from Manchuria to the Ukraine; and a possible third centre in central Africa in the region of the Great Lakes (see Figure 5.8). All these plague foci are in grassland areas which are only partially farmed or grazed; an environment

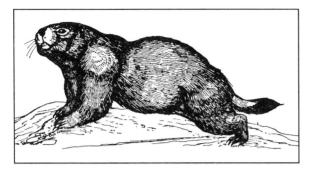

Figure 6.2 A Manchurian marmot.

well suited to colonies of marmots (see Figure 6.2), susliks (ground squirrels) and other burrowing rodents. And it was from one of these foci that the bacillus set out on its long journey. Which is the original focus and how did the bacillus come to spread from there to rodents and to human beings around the world?

There is considerable dispute among medical historians over these issues. McNeill believes that the Himalayas were the original home of the bacillus and that it has since spread via human activities, such as warfare, improved transport and increased trade. On this theory, it is social change which has destroyed the traditional ecological balances and allowed the infection to rampage beyond its traditional home.

☐　What evidence is there that human activities triggered off the three pandemics?

■　We saw earlier how traditional accounts link the appearance of the second pandemic to Tartar armies near the Black Sea. And shipping clearly played a major role in bringing the plague to Italy, Marseille, Melcombe (Dorset) and the Americas.

Serious criticisms can, however, be made of what the Canadian historian, John Norris, has called the 'ultimate reservoir' theory. First, the natural or 'inveterate' foci have throughout historic times almost certainly been more widespread than McNeill allows. But more importantly, all along the vast southern borders of the foci there are more populous areas where plague has for centuries been endemic in its secondary rodent hosts, the rat population, and periodically epidemic in the human population — parts of Asia Minor, Egypt, Syria, Iraq and Iran, northern India, Burma and the western provinces of China. These areas have for centuries acted as buffers or filters for the plague-free regions beyond (see Figure 6.3).

In looking for an explanation of the sudden appearance of the major epidemics, we are therefore looking for a factor capable of destabilising the conditions within the plague foci; of penetrating the filters of the border zones; of launching the disease into the non-immune regions beyond;

and of doing so on three separate occasions. Much the most likely factor is the development, each time, of a new strain of the disease, produced by mutation, just as 'flu develops new forms in ape and other animal populations. The plague bacillus is known to mutate, though much more slowly than the 'flu viruses. In recent years, for instance, American doctors in Vietnam identified a new, mild, upper-respiratory form of plague in which sufferers acted unknowingly as carriers. Such a 'new strains' hypothesis seems to fit the actual facts of the three pandemics rather better than the population growth or improved transport factors of McNeill's thesis.

A form of biological explanation may also work best in accounting for the disappearance of plague from many areas of the world which it had ravaged for centuries. A great variety of answers have been suggested to this problem; some have appealed to social changes, others to changes within the biological world. In the case of eighteenth-century Europe, all kinds of things have been suggested. Among all the possible factors — better quarantine, cleaner bodies (more soap), cleaner clothes (cotton underwear), more nutritious food (sugar and potatoes), new brick houses (more rat-resistant), the replacement of plague by a competitor (the bacillus responsible for tuberculosis), and the gradual replacement of the bold climbing black rat by the less sociable brown rat — the one which seems least subject to reservations is the development of a measure of long-term immunity among rodents. The long history of plague pandemics suggests that rodents living outside the inveterate foci, in the border zones and beyond, may have gradually (over the course of several centuries) developed some long-term resistance to the new strain of *Yersinia pestis*. The 'fireball'

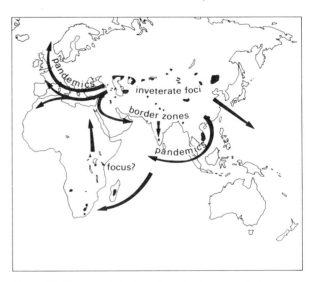

Figure 6.3 The spread of plague from the inveterate foci.

phenomenon, a violent epidemic which killed the remaining non-immune rats, might then indeed have left an immune population. Only in the optimum environmental conditions of the inveterate foci and in rodent species perfectly adapted as hosts would the microorganism survive in its most virulent form. There is one problem with this thesis. The development of this resistance has not so far been observed in the period since the beginning of the third pandemic. But, on the basis of the past history of the microorganism, this is not necessarily to be expected by this stage.

Given the speculative nature of this explanation, not everyone shares the biological point of view which stresses the role of mutation and resistance. The historian Paul Slack has warned against 'the temptation to attribute past events to one biological factor for which there is no historical evidence'. But, of course, there could *never* be any direct biological evidence: the microorganisms and the organs they attacked have gone for ever, and contemporary observers like Procopius and Boccaccio were quite unable to record for posterity the kinds of information we would need to reconstruct them. That does not mean they were not significant, nor that the evidence which does survive (like brick houses) *must* be significant. It is like an Agatha Christie detective story in which we conclude that the parlour maid must be the murderer because she is the only member of the household who is not dead, and we cannot interrogate the butler because he has committed suicide. The history of disease will always be more difficult to write than the history of pots and pans.

Traditional medical explanations

The plague bacillus was not discovered until 1894; the role of the flea emerged only in 1898. How did medical theory explain plague until that point? To examine this question, let us begin by looking at a passage from Daniel Defoe's *A Journal of the Plague Year*, set in the Great Plague of London in 1665. Defoe had lived through this as a child and, with the return of the plague to Marseille and Toulon in 1720, he wrote this detailed fictional account, based on a great variety of medieval and contemporary records and reminiscences, much of which centres around the problems of explaining this devastating and baffling phenomenon.

> ... I ought to leave a farther Remark for the use of Posterity, concerning the Manner of Peoples infecting one another; namely, that it was not the sick People only, from whom the Plague was immediately receiv'd by others that were sound, but THE WELL. . . .By the Well, I mean such as had received the Contagion, and had it really upon them, and in their Blood, yet did not show the Consequences of it in their Countenances, nay even were not sensible of it

> themselves, as many were not for several Days . . . . Now it was impossible to know these People, nor did they sometimes, as I have said, know themselves to be infected . . . .

> ... none knows when, or where, or how they may have received the Infection, or from whom. This I take to be the Reason, which makes so many People talk of the Air being corrupted and infected, and that they need not be cautious of whom they converse with, for that the Contagion was in the Air. I have seen them in strange Agitations and Surprises on this Account, 'I have never come near any infected Body!' says the disturbed Person, 'I have Convers'd with none, but sound healthy People, and yet I have gotten the Distemper!' 'I am sure I am struck from Heaven,' says another, and he falls to the serious Part; again the first goes on exclaiming, 'I have come near no Infection, or any infected Person, I am sure it is in the Air; We draw in Death when we breath...' [However] I must be allowed to believe, that no one in this whole Nation ever receiv'd the sickness or Infection, but who receiv'd it in the ordinary Way of Infection from some Body, or the Cloaths, or touch, or stench of some Body that was infected before. (Defoe, 1902, pp.215–20)

Before the late nineteenth century and the development of germ theory, there were two main theories of epidemic disease — those of *miasma* and *contagion* — both of which are implicitly referred to in Defoe's account. The miasmatic theory derived from the Hippocratic notion of a balance between human beings and their environment and, in the Hippocratic writings, epidemics were thought to be due to changed weather conditions. By the Middle Ages, the theory had changed a little. By then there was general agreement that it was an alteration or corruption of the atmosphere which engendered disease. The Greek word from which miasma derives means a stain, and the air was thought to be polluted by noxious exhalations from putrefying organic matter or stagnant water. These miasmas altered the body's humours, thus producing disease. This was the theory held by the nineteenth-century sanitary reformers who strove to clean up slums, lay down sewers and purify the water after the great cholera epidemic of 1831. Florence Nightingale, for example, was a fervent advocate of miasmatic theory.

The rival doctrine of contagion was absent from classical medical writings, though it is to be found in the Old Testament. In many respects, this is the ancestor of modern germ theory. Miasmatic ideas, however, dominated the medical analysis of epidemic disease until the late nineteenth century, though contagion formed a strong rival tradition. Its key early advocate was the Italian doctor, Girolamo Fracastoro (1478–1553) who believed in the existence of 'seminaria', or seeds, minute infective agents responsible for specific diseases which were both transmissible and, so he believed, self-propagating.

Neither theory worked perfectly and many felt that both might have something in them. Leprosy was generally taken to be contagious, malaria to be miasmatic. (The word malaria literally means 'bad air'.) Likewise, although miasmatic theories were generally more influential, the institution of quarantine was based on contagionist doctrine.

◻ Before the beginning of this century, no one knew anything of the role of rodents, fleas or bacilli in the generation of plague epidemics. All that was known was the different forms of plague and the impossibility of containing the disease. What sorts of difficulty do you think miasmatic and contagionist theories encountered when they tried to explain the spread of plague? (Re-reading Defoe will help.)

■ Plague, in its two very distinct forms, presented obvious difficulties for analysis. Observations of pneumonic plague epidemics lent support to the contagonist argument, but the interrelationship between pneumonic and bubonic plague, and the puzzling ability of bubonic plague to jump quarantine lines and penetrate boarded-up houses, seemed to many observers only to be explicable in terms of some odourless and invisible miasma.

Plague therefore remained a central issue in a fierce, at times embittered, academic controversy between miasmatists and contagonists until the very end of the nineteenth century. Defoe, writing in 1722, was a rather sceptical contagonist, but Charles Creighton, writing his *History of Epidemics in Britain* in 1894, still the standard work, was a miasmatist. Die-hard miasmatists were writing letters to academic journals long after Yersin's and Kitasato's discoveries were accepted.

The social and economic impact of plague

Now that we have reviewed the explanations of plague in some detail, let us turn to examine its social and economic impact. Consider first its effect on people of different social classes.

In his account of the 1655–66 plague in the *History and Antiquities of Eyam*, published in 1842, a local historian called Wood says of the inhabitants: 'The most wealthy of them, who were but few in number, had fled early in the Spring with the greatest precipitation. Some few others having means, fled to the neighbouring hills.' (Bradley, 1977, p.65) Wood was writing 150 years after the event and relying only on anecdotal evidence. Nevertheless, given the patchiness of plague outbreaks, the story does suggest that

those who could afford to flee may possibly have suffered rather less. As we have already seen, Boccaccio's work, *The Decameron*, is a collection of tales supposedly told by members of the Florentine aristocracy who were residing in the countryside to escape from the plague. And the Scottish chronicler James of Fordun, who estimated a one-third total mortality, thought that the nobles escaped lightly in the first epidemic of 1348–49.

◻ What other reason might there be for a possible difference in the effect of plague on different social classes?

■ We saw in Chapter 4 that in 1831 cholera struck much harder among the poor. Bad housing, poor nutrition, polluted water, and the lack of sewers all seemed to increase the chances of suffering that particular infection.

So there are several reasons for thinking that the richer members of society may have got off more lightly during the great plague epidemics. How can we check whether this is true? One problem is that most of the objective evidence from the fourteenth century consists of records of taxpayers, rent-payers and office-holders drawn up by manorial lords and by royal and ecclesiastical authorities. This can reveal something about the numbers of better-off people who died but tells us little of the mortality among the poor. The question of the incidence of the Black Death and later plague epidemics among the various social classes has therefore been much debated, the inadequacy of the sources making it possible for opposing points of view to be held on the basis of the same body of evidence. The Titchfield tenants, with their 60 per cent mortality in 1348–49, are an example: were they wealthier than and therefore healthier than labourers, or poorer and therefore more vulnerable than freeholders?

One source with which we can compare the tenant mortality are the lists of parish priests which bishops kept. These show very heavy mortality among priests. In the deanery of Southampton just west of Titchfield the mortality was 66 per cent, very similar to that among the tenants in Titchfield. In the whole diocese of Winchester, priest mortality was nearly 50 per cent, the highest in England; but even in the diocese of York, in which it is supposed that the disease began to lose some of its virulence, it was over 40 per cent. The evidence has once again been interpreted in different ways. Were the priests, though poor, still better fed than other poor people, or did they, while devotedly performing their priestly duties, contract plague more easily?

For the highest social class, the nobility who held land directly from the King, and whose deaths were reported to him, the American historian J.C. Russell (1948) has calculated a 27 per cent mortality in 1348–49. Perhaps the

Scottish chronicler, James of Fordun, was right in saying that they got off lightly. On the other hand, all it may reveal is that the nobility, whose manor houses were scattered evenly all over the country, give us a better indication of the national mortality than the Titchfield tenants, exposed to a pneumonic epidemic, or the priests made vulnerable by their occupation. Moreover, if the nobles did escape lightly in the first epidemic, they may have paid for their escape in a relative lack of immunity in the second epidemic of 1361–62. This epidemic, called by some chroniclers 'the children's plague' because of their high mortality, was called by others the 'nobleman's plague'. Guy de Chauliac was among those who noticed high mortality among the wealthy in Europe at that time, and J.C. Russell's 25 per cent figure for the English nobility in this second epidemic is indeed higher than our estimate of 20 per cent for ordinary tenants at Titchfield.

There are therefore some difficulties in being certain about the matter. Overall, however, there does not seem to have been much difference in social class mortality. Plague apparently struck regardless of living conditions, nutrition, or the possession of country estates.

So that is the first social effect to consider: the relatively uniform impact of plague on people of different social classes. Now let us turn to examine the way it affected the behaviour of those who survived. Here, once again, is a description from Defoe of the Great Plague of London of 1665:

> . . . after the Funerals became so many, that People could not toll the Bell, Mourn, or Weep, or wear Black for one another, as they did before; no, nor so much as make Coffins for those that died; so after a while the fury of the Infection appeared to be so encreased, that in short, they shut up no Houses at all; it seem'd enough that all the Remedies of that Kind had been used till they were found fruitless, and that the Plague spread itself with an irresistible Fury, so that, as the Fire the succeeding Year [the Great Fire of London, 1666], spread itself and burnt with such Violence, that the Citizens in Despair, gave over their Endeavours to extinguish it, so in the Plague, it came at last to such Violence that the People sat still looking at one another, and seem'd quite abandon'd to Despair; whole Streets seem'd to be desolated, and not to be shut up only, but to be emptied of their Inhabitants; Doors were left open, Windows stood shattering with the Wind in empty Houses, for want of people to shut them: In a Word, People began to give up themselves to their Fears, and to think that all regulations and Methods were in vain, and that there was nothing to be hoped for, but an universal Desolation . . . . (Defoe, 1902, p.193)

It is difficult for most of us, currently shielded as we are by all the resources of modern society from extreme pain and the presence of death, to comprehend the reactions of our ancestors to plague epidemics like those of the second pandemic. Not surprisingly, many people's first reaction was religious; supernatural as well as natural explanations were involved:

> . . . I looked, and behold a pale horse: and the name that sat on him was Death, and Hell followed with him. And power was given unto them over the fourth part of the earth, to kill with sword, and with hunger, and with death, and with the beasts of the earth . . . and no man was able to enter into the temple, till the seven plagues of the seven angels were fulfilled.
> (Revelations 6: 8)

The Black Death itself, and the successive epidemics of the second pandemic, seemed to many to be unfolding these prophecies of the Book of Revelations (something that is vividly portrayed in Bergman's film *The Seventh Seal*, 1956). To them, plague was an Act of God, sent to punish both individuals and whole societies for their transgressions. Their main hope of relief lay, therefore, not in medicine but in religious acts.

The severity of the first impact of plague seems to have provoked a particularly extreme form of religious penitence, the flagellant movement of 1348–49, during which groups of men and women wandered from village to village beating one another with cruelly designed whips. The transgressions for which plague was a punishment might also be supposed to be the work of evil spirits residing in certain individuals or groups, which could be driven out only by torture or burning. One result was a vicious outbreak of anti-semitism throughout much of Europe during 1348–49. The first massacres took place in southern France and Spain in the spring of 1348. Then in the autumn, in Basle in Switzerland, whole communities of Jews were burned alive in locked buildings or pits — a practice that spread to Germany and the Low Countries before being stamped out towards the end of 1349 by governments afraid of anarchy and civil disorder.

In addition, in the early stages of many epidemics there were episodes of panic-stricken flight and the desertion of homes and properties. A number of contemporary observers record instances of individuals and whole communities drinking, dancing, singing and indulging in sexual excesses. 'Eat, drink and be merry, for tomorrow you may die.' Harmless hedonism then sometimes merged into rape, looting, purposeless violence and other symptoms of a society in a state of collapse. One form of behaviour, called by some historians the dancing fever, seems to have been peculiar to the fifteenth century. Agonised and delirious running, mentioned by writers like

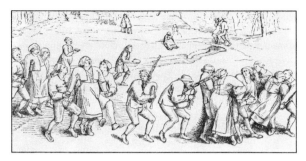

Figure 6.4 Medieval sufferers from dancing mania on a pilgrimage accompanied by musicians.

Procopius and Defoe, was a physical symptom of plague itself, but other instances of frenzied groups of dancers moving from village to village, collapsing and sometimes dying of exhaustion, suggest imitative mass hysteria rather than any purely physical condition (see Figure 6.4). The later stages of epidemics also, as Defoe records, sometimes saw a different mood, of helplessness and apathetic despair.

Events such as these, however terrible, were short-term. What of the longer-term effects? Memories of plague lingered in the consciousness of European peoples for many centuries, sometimes in half-concealed ways. The nursery rhyme 'Ring-a-ring a roses, a pocket full of posies, a-tishoo, a-tishoo, all fall down' is, for example, thought to refer to bubonic plague.

   □ Why?

   ■ 'Ring-a-ring a roses' may represent the buboes with their characteristic circular shape; posies were small bunches of flowers used to ward off miasmas; 'a-tishoo, a-tishoo' could be the sneezing associated with the pneumonic form; 'all fall down' would then need no interpretation.

We may have inherited many other things besides rhymes from this experience. Some historians feel that as well as religious change, plague also produced some major *economic effects*. Figure 6.5 combines an estimate of changes in the English population from 1250 to 1750 (the

curving line) with a further estimate of changes in the wages paid to craftsmen during this period (the shaded blocks).

   □ Examine the changes in the curving line (the population) during this period. What does this suggest about the long-term impact of the second pandemic? (Population figures are given on the right-hand side of the figure.)

   ■ That it made the population fall from around 5.5 million in 1350 to a low of only just over 2 million in 1450. Only in the eighteenth century, the period when plague had disappeared from England, did the population attain its previous level.

There are many problems with this analysis. There are major difficulties in estimating the size of the population at this time and there is a very considerable difference between the various estimates that have been made. Figure 6.6 illustrates this for the period 1086–1525. The bottom line represents the smallest estimate that seems currently plausible; the top line gives the largest plausible figure. As you can see, these are big differences. Nevertheless, there is general agreement, whatever estimate is chosen, that there was a dramatic fall in population after the arrival of the Black Death. This might not all be necessarily due to plague. Some have argued that the population of England was already over-large in relation to its food resources and that famine was the cause of much of this decline. Others have thought that infectious diseases besides plague also had a major effect. Yet others have pointed to the long-term climatic deterioration that also began in the fourteenth century. All these factors may also have played a part. Nevertheless, the detailed evidence that we looked at in Chapter 5, the studies of the effects of plague in particular towns and villages, does suggest that plague must have had a major role in the long-term decline of both the English and the wider European populations.

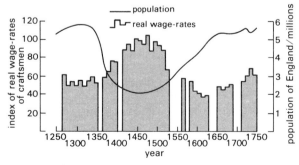

Figure 6.5 Changes in (a) English population, (b) craftsmen's real wage-rates; 1250–1750. (Hatcher 1977, p.71)

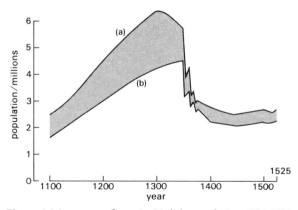

Figure 6.6 Long-term flows in English population 1086–1525, showing the ranges between plausible estimates. (Hatcher 1977, p.71)

☐ Now go back to Figure 6.5, which compared changes in population with changes in craftsmen's wages. (The scale for wages is on the left-hand side of the figure.) What do these estimates suggest about the effect of changes in population upon wages?

■ As the population fell, wages rose. Eventually, when the population started to rise again, wages fell back to around their old level.

Estimating wages presents as many problems as does estimating population or the effects of plague on that population. Nonetheless, many historians believe that, by reducing the population of Europe by one-third to a half, plague greatly improved the living standards of the survivors. Some also believe that the combination of devastating disease and major economic change fundamentally transformed European society. In 1927 the German historian, E. Friedell, went so far as to argue that 'the year of the conception of modern man was the year 1348, the year of the Black Death' (Friedell, 1927, p.62). On this argument, the only sufferers from plague, from an economic point of view, were the large land-owners who had produced foodstuffs for the pre-plague market. Everyone else enjoyed higher living standards. As a result they bought more consumer goods of all kinds — non-essential foods, pots and pans, clothes, ornaments; trade increased; and the merchant classes and those aristocrats with trading interests prospered. These then were the people who paid for the buildings, sculptures, paintings and books of the Italian Renaissance; who bought the new kinds of books produced on printing presses; who supported the Protestant churches during the Reformation; who put up the money for voyages of discovery to the Americas and the Indies; and so on. None of this would have happened (it is said) had Europe not suffered disease on a massive scale. Many historians disagree strongly with arguments like those of Friedell. It is unlikely that we shall ever be certain about these matters. The rise of Europe no doubt had many other causes. Plague may nevertheless have had a significant effect.

Conclusions

The principal theme of this course is the biosocial nature of health and disease. We cannot fully understand any disease unless we approach it simultaneously from the perspectives of both the biological and the social sciences. Homilies like this are, however, much easier to say than to put into practice. Every discipline likes to cling to what it knows and to believe that it has all the answers, or at least all the really important ones. There may also be other factors that prejudice us in favour of one sort of approach and lead us to ignore the other. McNeill makes the following argument:

We all want human experience to make sense, and historians cater to this universal demand by emphasising elements in the past that are calculable, definable, and, often, controllable as well. Epidemic disease, when it did become decisive in peace or in war, ran counter to the effort to make the past intelligible. Historians consequently played such episodes [as the Black Death] down. (McNeill, 1979, p.12)

Many historians and other social scientists have, therefore, tended to minimise the impact of disease on human history and instead sought answers in population growth or economic and technological change*. Even McNeill prefers to stress human elements as the key factor in the outbreak of the three pandemics, whereas a biological factor — the emergence of a new strain — seems a more plausible explanation.

We should also not forget that, even though plague is currently held at bay, some other microorganisms still pose a major threat to human life. Not only are they the major cause of mortality in the Third World, but even the West can still be ravaged by a new epidemic. The great 'flu pandemic of 1918–19 is this century's classic example. Like the Black Death, this pandemic swept indiscriminately through urban and rural communities, through the crowded cities of the industrialised West, the peasant communities of Asia, and then to remote societies all over the world, reportedly wiping out the populations of some small Pacific islands. The number of deaths in England and Wales was estimated as 150 000 and throughout the world as 20 million, many more than died in Europe during the Black Death, though of course in a much larger population. More recent 'flu epidemics have claimed fewer lives — some 7 000–8 000, for instance, in the United Kingdom in 1961, 1970 and 1976 — and it has been suggested by some that this has been the result of improved social conditions and of better nutrition. Once again, however, it seems more plausible that this was due to a change in the virulence of the disease.

☐ Why does this seem more plausible?

■ If the 1918–19 epidemic swept indiscriminately through advanced and primitive societies, its virulence must have had little relationship to health and nutrition factors. And if it were to return today, despite continued improvements in living standards, it might still have the same effect.

---

* These matters will be explored further in *The Health of Nations*. The Open University (1985) *The Health of Nations*, The Open University Press. (U205 *Health and Disease*, Book III).

More recently, though on a much smaller scale, there have been outbreaks of several newly identified infectious diseases: Marburg 'green monkey' disease (1967), Lassa fever (1969), Legionnaire's disease (1976) and, most recently of all, AIDS.

In summary, for all that modern society has made enormous economic, scientific and social advances, there are certain respects in which the life of the human species may still be precariously balanced. We have not obtained complete control over the microorganisms which devastated our ancestors, nor are we ever likely to do so. The moral of the story is that we should always pay close attention to what are sometimes termed the *exogenous* factors in human life, those factors that lie outside the human social process. As McNeill warns, there is sometimes a tendency to look solely for social explanations, to select the *endogenous* factors, those internal to human society, and ignore the others.

Having said this, the theme of the course is still that of the biosocial nature of human existence. The biological interpretation of the three pandemics that has been put forward here used to be popular once upon a time, fell into disrepute and only regained popularity in recent years, and may change again. Moreover, even if one accepts it, there are still crucial ways in which the transmission of plague around the globe has depended on factors endogenous to human social life: wars, trade, steamships and the like. Plague is merely at one end of a biosocial continuum.

In Chapters 7–9 we go on to explore the other end of this continuum: the way in which some medical conditions may be largely the product not of biological but of social factors. Even at this other extreme, however, the same general lesson holds true. However powerful social forces may be, or appear to be, one should never entirely neglect the biological end of the spectrum. The understanding of health and disease, requires a fully biosocial approach.

Objectives for Chapter 6

When you have studied this chapter, you should be able to:

6.1 Describe the causes and course of plague pandemics in terms of both endogenous (e.g. transport) and exogenous (e.g. mutation) factors and the necessity for a biosocial approach to the problem.

6.2 Discuss traditional miasmatic and contagionist explanations of epidemics of infectious disease.

6.3 Describe the religious, class and economic impact of plague on Europe.

Questions for Chapter 6

1 (*Objective 6.1*) 'Within a decade of its arrival in Hong Kong [1894] all the important seaports of the world experienced outbreaks of the dread disease.' (McNeill, 1979, p.144). Does this suggest that the third pandemic was due to endogenous or exogenous factors?

2 (*Objective 6.2*) Turn back to the quotation from Boccaccio in Chapter 5 (p.43). What theories about the origin of plague are mentioned there, either explicitly or implicitly?

3 (*Objective 6.3*) 'The plague not only depopulates and kills, it gnaws the moral stamina and frequently destroys it entirely, thus the sudden demoralisation of Roman society from the period of Mark Antony may be explained by the Oriental plague ... in such epidemics the best were invariably carried off and the survivors deteriorated morally. Times of plague are always those in which the bestial and diabolical side of human nature gains the upper hand.' (B.G. Neibuhr, quoted in Ziegler, 1970, p.267).

Is Niebuhr's pessimistic view of the destructive effects of plague correct?

7
Hysterectomy: a surgical epidemic?

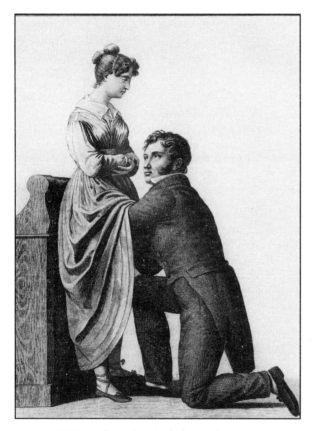

Figure 7.1 A traditional method of vaginal examination.

In the *Index Medicus*, a monthly index of all new articles appearing in medical journals throughout the world, 'hysterectomy', the subject of this chapter, comes immediately before 'hysteria', the subject of our final case study. The words sound similar yet mean something rather different. 'Hysterectomy' is the surgical removal of the womb. 'Hysteria' is defined rather formidably by *The Concise Oxford Dictionary* as 'Psychoneurosis with anaesthesia, convulsions, etc., and usu. with disturbance of moral and intellectual faculties; uncontrolled or morbid excitement'. Both stem from the Greek work 'hustera', meaning womb. Hysterectomy is a relatively new medical word — the surgical removal of the womb has been possible only since the nineteenth century. But hysteria is one of the oldest diagnostic terms in Western medicine, going back to Hippocratic times (*c*.400 BC) and beyond. To the Greeks, hysteria was a condition suffered exclusively by women — its origins lay with the womb; hence the name. Indeed, it was only in the nineteenth century that this ancient belief was abandoned and alternative theories of hysteria proposed.

There are some other important links between hysteria and hysterectomy. Each condition largely or wholly concerns women. Each is an example of a possible epidemic. Each also reveals something about the nature of academic and public debate and something about the changing role of medicine. For although there are many parallels between the first era of therapeutic nihilism and that through which we are passing today, there is at least one strikingly new criticism of medicine: the charge that it acts as an instrument of *social control*. According to this criticism, the panoply of modern medicine — its diagnostic techniques, surgery and drugs — is used in the interests of the powerful and the strong. Critics vary in precisely whom they accuse. For some it is the State whose interests are ultimately served; for others, it is the interests of the young versus those of the aged, or those of the middle classes versus those of the working classes. Of all these critiques, that made by women has received most prominence. For many feminist critics, medicine serves the interests of the male gender. According to these critics, this is not a particularly modern phenomenon. For them, Western medicine has always served men rather than women, has largely excluded women from the élite medical occupations and has consistently treated female patients in a demeaning and often brutal fashion. Men have used medicine, psychiatry and surgery to further their own control over women. The characterisation of women's anatomy, physiology and mental state is far from the impartial, scientific study implied by the Whig history of medical science, or so it is argued.

The next three chapters, which focus on hysteria and hysterectomy, serve as a general introduction to the feminist critique and to some of the counter-arguments that have also been made. Three points should be noted here. First, feminism, the analysis and critique of women's social role, comes in many different forms, some more radical than others. Second, since this debate is of such wide-reaching significance and touches on almost every aspect of health, disease and medicine, we shall return to it throughout the course. Many of the arguments raised here for the first time will be dealt with in more detail elsewhere. Finally, these three chapters also introduce some of the basic issues in studying medical treatments and mental illness; here too there are many controversies and many problems still to be solved. And here also a more detailed analysis of these matters must wait; this is merely an hors-d'oeuvre.

Hysterectomy: a history

Earlier in this book, we considered the Whig approach to the history of medicine, which centres around the 'onward and upward' view of medical science. Hysterectomy, too, can be seen in this fashion. In 1853, Burnham performed the first 'successful' hysterectomy. However, of the fifteen patients on whom he tried this procedure, only three survived. Given this mortality rate, the operation was long confined to extreme conditions: to cancer of the uterus and to obstetric catastrophes such as uncontrolled bleeding and uterine rupture. Hysterectomy was an operation of last resort.

☐   What might have changed all this? And when?
■   Lister's development of antisepsis in the 1860s, though this did not have its full effect until the end of the century, and even later.

With improved anaesthetics, antisepsis and, later, asepsis, the fall in the mortality rate was dramatic. Whereas Burnham lost 80 per cent of his patients, the current mortality rate for hysterectomy is around 0.02 per cent.

Despite this fall, most surgeons continued for a long time to be highly cautious in their use of hysterectomy. The criteria for the operation, or indications as they are technically known, were sharply circumscribed. Hysterectomy remained a *mandatory* rather than an *elective* operation, in other words it was to be performed only when the patient's condition was grave. Conditions which did not threaten a woman's life, however painful or distressing they might be, were to be treated by other means. Here, for example, from a book published in 1898, is a discussion of *menorrhagia*, or excessive bleeding, a condition which is sometimes linked to 'fibroids' (benign uterine tumours which can cause extreme pain and major and prolonged bleeding during menstruation — today the most common indication for hysterectomy):

> The menstrual periods under the best of circumstances are a great impediment to a woman, but when the flow becomes profuse and perhaps irregular in its appearance, her life may become a burden to her. Full-bloodedness, intemperance, too frequent child-bearing, tumours and bad labours, excite congestion of the pelvic organs and are the chief causes of menorrhagia.
>
> TREATMENT Ladies who are full-blooded require to live temperately. Often to get rid of the excess of blood, Nature finds an outlet by increasing the loss at monthly periods. This should not be rashly checked. Treatment should be directed to the cause of the plethora. A spare diet with little meat, and tea or coffee or milk-and-water to drink, is best suited to such a case. Alcohol is always highly prejudicial and should be sternly forbidden.
>
> [The following treatments are then recommended where necessary] potassium bromide; diluted sulphuric acid; ergot; juice of four lemons or a wine-glassful of vinegar; hydrastis canadensis; arsenic; aletris cordial; sulphur waters such as those found at Harrogate; and potassium iodide. (The Chemist and Druggist, 1898, pp.120–22)

☐   How serious a condition is menorrhagia according to this account?
■   Certainly not life-threatening but definitely serious, for it can make a woman's life 'become a burden to her'.

Surgery does not receive a mention in this discussion but, over the next few decades, surgeons gradually relaxed their criteria for hysterectomy. The drug treatments suggested above were not particularly effective; hysterectomy, however, worked, and it came to be used both for menorrhagia and for a variety of other non-fatal uterine disorders. Indeed, the mortality from hysterectomy is now so low that, even where the womb is not diseased, some modern gynaecologists have urged that *every* woman can benefit from the operation. The American gynaecologist Ralph C. Wright argued thus in 1969: 'The uterus has but one function: reproduction. After the last planned pregnancy, the uterus becomes a useless, bleeding, symptom-producing, potentially cancer-bearing organ and should be removed . . .' (Wright, 1969. p.562)

In the last 100 years, hysterectomy has, therefore, moved from being an operation of the last resort to something that is urged, by some doctors, on all women, regardless of whether they are actually ill or not. Indeed, on current trends, more than half of all American women will have the operation at some time in their lives, as will one in five British women. Hysterectomy is now the most common of all forms of major surgery. But, as we shall now see, it is also — and for this very same reason — one of the most controversial of all operations.

The unnecessary hysterectomy

The modern campaign against the use of hysterectomy on such a wide scale may be said to have begun on 29 October 1945. The Chicago Lying-in Hospital was celebrating its fiftieth anniversary and, as part of this, one of its gynaecologists, Norman Miller, had been asked to give a paper to various assembled dignatories. His address was most unusual for such occasions, for its title was 'Hysterectomy: Therapeutic Necessity or Surgical Racket?' Through examining their records, Miller had studied all the hysterectomies conducted in ten hospitals in the first four months of 1945. He noted that 10 per cent of these women had originally sought medical care for 'secondary' reasons such as fatigue, irritability, nervousness and headache; 17 per cent had no physical complaint to make — 'an interesting observation since most patients submitted to major surgery usually have a reason for seeking medical care'; in 19 per cent no disease of the pelvic organs was revealed by pelvic examination; and in 31 per cent of all cases pathological examination of the uterus following hysterectomy revealed no evidence of disease — a finding which he called 'stunning' and 'startling' and which he explained through a new gynaecological concept: 'the remunerative or hip-pocket hysterectomy'. He concluded with the following words: 'If what we have observed in this look behind the scenes is confirmed by future studies, then we may be sure that, when the curtain rises, we shall witness a tragedy, painful and far-reaching in its implications.' (Miller, 1946, p.810)

☐ What are the key differences between Norman Miller and Ralph C. Wright as regards:
 (a) the indications for hysterectomy?
 (b) the motivation of gynaecologists who perform very large numbers of hysterectomies?

■ (a) Miller maintains that hysterectomy is justified only where there is uterine disease; Wright thinks the womb should be removed once a woman no longer intends to use it for reproduction.

(b) Miller thinks that some hysterectomies are performed because surgeons have a financial incentive to perform them; Wright sees them as simply offering a service to women.

These two fiercely opposed positions can be linked to the traditional battle within surgery between the 'conservatives' and the 'liberals', terms which refer to their surgical policy, not to their wider politics. The conservatives take a cautious approach and treat surgery as a highly invasive therapy. They wish to 'conserve the flesh' wherever possible. To them, the 'liberals' or 'radicals', who believe in more radical or heroic surgery and in the general therapeutic value of cutting, are sometimes rash or irresponsible. To the radicals the cautious surgeon is hardly a surgeon at all. Surgery, by its very nature, demands great self-confidence. Does the cautious surgeon 'really like getting his fingers inside people'? Will he hesitate where he should operate?

The battle between the different schools is normally waged in private, though, for a variety of reasons, American surgeons are sometimes more forthright. One spokesman for the conservative view, and a future president of the American College of Surgeons, wrote in 1922: 'There are regrettably some unconscionable pot-hunters who will operate on anybody that will hold still. Every hospital should eliminate that kind of man.' (Smith, 1922, p.820) His critique was not, however, based on research. Miller's 1946 attack was — and was given in a public forum. His findings were reported in the *Reader's Digest* and the *Ladies Home Journal*, and they began a public debate in North America that has continued to this day. Since Miller's paper, further such inquiries have been produced, not only by gynaecologists, but also by the Teamsters' Union (the American truck-drivers' union), which claimed that 30 per cent of the hysterectomies in their study were unnecessary; by insurance companies; and in 1974 by Congress itself.

Following such reports and concerned about the rising costs of health care, several US states and insurance companies have made a serious attempt to lower the rate of hysterectomy, either through systematic inspection of surgeons' records, or else through making a second medical opinion compulsory. Such attempts have met with only mixed success. Overall, the American hysterectomy rate has continued to rise throughout the 1970s, though at a considerably slower pace than it did in the previous decade.

Since the British hysterectomy rate is less than half that of the United States, there has not been the same public outcry against the operation. Nevertheless, there are many people who think that even the British rate is far too high. Angela Phillips and Jill Rakusen (1978, p.184), the authors of the British edition of a popular women's health handbook, *Our Bodies Ourselves*, state simply 'There are undoubtedly too many hysterectomies performed in this country', an opinion echoed by two British doctors, Joyce Leeson and Judith Gray (1978, p.141), also writing for a general audience, who comment critically on 'the shortcomings of the take-it-all-away approach'. To perform major surgery on one-fifth of all women certainly requires detailed examination and justification.

Is hysterectomy prophylactic?

One of R.C. Wright's major arguments for the general use of hysterectomy was that is was *prophylactic*; that is, not only would it save all women from the discomforts of menstruation, and some women from the pain of menorrhagia, but also that it would remove the fear and the actuality of future disease, particularly of uterine and cervical cancer (the cervix is normally removed along with the uterus). The possibility of cancer frightens many of us. Something that will remove that fear, at least for some kinds of cancer, seems well worth doing. But is it? Does hysterectomy actually lengthen women's lives?

☐   In what way might hysterectomy possibly shorten women's lives?

■   Some women die following surgery. No operation is completely safe, and all treatments have 'side-effects', some of which are noxious, even fatal.

Statisticians have compared how many women die following such surgery with the number who might otherwise have been expected to die from uterine and cervical cancers. They have also tried to take into account the recent finding from two studies that suggest that hysterectomy may increase some women's vulnerability to coronary heart disease. Weighing these various costs and benefits is extremely difficult. However, the most recent studies suggest that R.C. Wright may be right; hysterectomy does appear to lengthen the average woman's life. But it does so, at least on these calculations, by only a trivial amount, a few months — much the same period of time that is needed to convalesce after the operation.

Against the patient's will

So far we have looked at the criticisms of hysterectomy made by sceptical doctors and statisticians and by those who pay some of the financial costs. But patients, too, have had their own complaints to make. Here, for example, is an extract from a letter in the magazine *Good Housekeeping*, which had earlier published an article about one woman's experience of hysterectomy:

I couldn't agree with anything more than with what Val Wilmer says. I am almost glad to know that it wasn't just that I had been singled out for such off-hand treatment. After several years of cervical erosions I was admitted for the seventh time to my usual London teaching hospital for a 24-hour job of cauterisation. However, this time I saw a new doctor who decided immediately that this was a case for hysterectomy. I said that this was a great surprise and that I had only come prepared for 24 hours and not 10 days; that I had a family to think of. I was told that I had one hour to think the matter over while he finished his rounds. I then agreed or vacated the bed because no-one was twisting my arm. In great distress because I couldn't contact my lorry driver husband I agreed and I feel bitter that at the age of 35 I had to make a decision that has certainly changed my life. I was told that if I went home I would be back within a year with more trouble than I had bargained for, although I never found out what he meant, and that I could then wait a further year on the waiting list. I felt that I had no choice at all . . . . Now after 11 months I have been seeing a psychiatrist for the last two for severe depression, which not only affects me but my whole family . . . I do feel physically much better but mentally I do not. (Cass, 1982, p.40)

And here is an extract from a book about American gynaecology by a feminist sociologist, Diana Scully, based on observation of surgical practice in two hospitals:

The sales pitch used by residents [trainees] at both hospitals was remarkably similar; in some cases the very same words were used. The resident opened by moving from a general problem for which a number of solutions, including doing nothing, were possible, to the solution that he was going to try to sell, usually a hysterectomy. The more supporting evidence that could be brought to bear on the problem, the more secure the resident was in his pitch. The pitch frequently began when a woman over the age of thirty-five requested birth control or permanent sterilisation in the form of a tubal ligation. If, in addition, the resident could locate evidence of some pathology, he would attempt to sell a hysterectomy . . . my observations indicated that clinic women were never advised of the relative dangers or rates of complication of the vaginal hysterectomy . . . when the pathology involved a fibroid, the "tumour" was presented in such a way that the woman would initially become alarmed. Later, when the resident assured her that fibroids weren't cancerous, the psychological impact had already been made. (Scully, 1980, pp.224–5)

The allegation here is that some surgeons, perhaps many, are so keen to perform hysterectomies that they are willing to bully women into the operation. Why should they wish to do this? Miller suggested that in private medicine doctors have a direct financial incentive. Scully argues that in American teaching hospitals there are also strong 'educational' grounds. In the United States, though not in the United Kingdom, trainee surgeons need to have done set numbers of particular operations in order to qualify. This might seem to guarantee a certain standard of technical competence, but it might also lead to some patients being unnecessarily submitted to surgery. Two Australian doctors, one of them a community physician, the other a gynaecologist, emphasise both these points, and add a third: 'Hysterectomy is one of the few major operations done by the gynaecologists, and pride, technical practice and financial incentive may generate a bias towards this treatment.' (Selwood and Wood, 1978, p.202)

□ British rates of hysterectomy are lower than those of either the United States or Australia. Is this fact compatible with the possible explanations of surgical motivation mentioned above?

■ Yes. Most British patients are seen in the National Health Service, not privately. So that removes the financial incentive. (Australian health services have been largely private.) Likewise, there is not the same pressure for British trainees to perform a set number of operations.

The radical feminist critique

The evidence cited above was that some women were being forced into operations they themselves did not want. Is there any reason to think that women are being singled out? Some doctors might, perhaps, do this to all patients. Consider the following arguments. First, although women have been training as doctors for more than 100 years, they are still greatly underrepresented, for one reason or another, in most areas of hospital practice. Even in obstetrics and gynaecology, more than 90 per cent of consultants are men. The expectations of the *Punch* cartoon of 1872 are still far from being fulfilled (see Figure 7.2). Second, consider gynaecologists' attitudes towards women. What are the possible motivations of men who specialise in the routine vaginal and uterine exploration of women? Male gynaecologists are in an extremely powerful position over a very intimate portion of women's lives and anatomy. One male American gynaecologist has said:

I wouldn't want most of my patients to realize what an ego trip I get from taking care of them, because there's something selfish about enjoying the fact that a lot of women are dependent on you ... I think there are some in the specialty who like to punish women.

Some doctors really get a kind of unconscious kick from seeing a woman in labour. There are some doctors who are very sadistic. (quoted in Daly, 1979, p.260)

Just as we may want to scrutinise the motives of contemporary male doctors a little more closely, feminist historians have argued that the Whig history of medicine omits certain characteristic male attitudes towards women. Here, for example, is a quotation from a nineteenth-century English physician, Robert Carter, who developed the first psychiatric theory of repression:

No-one who has realized the amount of moral evil wrought in girls ... whose prurient desires have been increased by Indian hemp and partially gratified by medical manipulation, can deny that remedy is worse than disease. I have seen young unmarried women, of the middle class of society, reduced by the constant use of the speculum, to the mental and moral

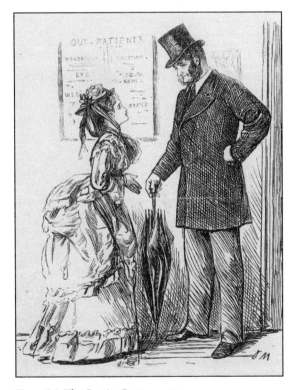

Figure 7.2 The Coming Race.
DOCTOR EVANGELINE By the bye, Mr Sawyer, are you engaged tomorrow afternoon? I have rather a ticklish operation to perform — an amputation, you know.
MR SAWYER I shall be very happy to do it for you.
DR EVANGELINE O, no, not *that*! But will you kindly come and administer the chloroform for me? (Punch, 1872)

constitutions of prostitutes; seeking to give themselves the same indulgence by the practice of solitary vice; and asking every medical practitioner ... to institute an examination of the sexual organs. (quoted in Scully, 1980, p.41)

This was written in 1853, shortly after the invention of the speculum (see Figure 7.3). (Some doctors, in fact, specialised solely in vaginal examination and were known as speculators.) The author is obviously worried about masturbation, an important Victorian preoccupation (both for boys and for girls, it was held to be dangerous, immoral or both). For girls the treatment of persistent masturbation even went so far as surgical removal of the clitoris — though this provoked a huge outcry and was performed on very few patients. Moreover, just as there are now fears about an epidemic of hysterectomy, the late nineteenth century saw a huge boom in oophorectomy (the removal of the ovaries) and a corresponding public campaign in which writers such as George Bernard Shaw and Emile Zola were major critics of contemporary gynaecological practice. To its adherents, however, oophorectomy was a remedy for all kinds of female ailments, both physical and mental:

Rohé, Manton and others have blazed the way; and what do they tell us? They tell us that castration pays; that patients are improved, some of them cured; that the moral sense of the patient is elevated, that she becomes tractable, orderly, industrious and cleanly .... My own experience in this line has been most happy. (quoted in Scully, 1980, p.51)

Such evidence seems quite powerful, but for some feminists we must go a good deal further than this. Their claim is that the whole development of science, including medical science, has been a peculiarly masculine affair. Some radical feminists have argued that folk medicine and folk healing were often the province of 'wise women', just as childbirth was the province of midwives. The rise of medicine excluded 'wise women' and replaced female midwives by male gynaecologists. On this argument, this replacement was often a violent procedure. Some who would in former times have been regarded as healers were now castigated and some perhaps even burned as witches. (Though a sixteenth-century male doctor in Germany, who disguised himself as a midwife in order to study childbirth, was himself burnt for impiety.)

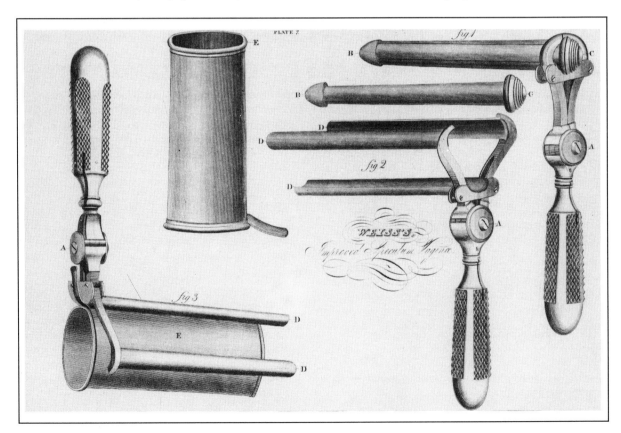

Figure 7.3 Victorian instruments for vaginal examination.

At the same time, according to the feminist historian Caroline Merchant (1982), the new medical and scientific approach to the world replaced the holistic, harmonious tradition with one which was simultaneously reductionist and centred on the domination and conquering of nature. Francis Bacon saw nature as female, the scientist's task to 'wrest her secrets from her' to 'penetrate her hidden parts', to strip aside her 'veil of secrecy', to leave nature naked and exposed to view, to force her unwilling surrender of hidden truth. For Merchant, these metaphors of the rape of nature profoundly colour the ways in which science, including medical science, has developed from the seventeenth to the twentieth century. She holds that this male knowledge affects all scientific practice and understanding of the world. On this argument, male medicine's treatment of women, as exemplified by both hysterectomy and hysteria, becomes explicable as part of male science's attempt to dominate a (female) nature.

The American radical feminist, and ex-nun, Mary Daly takes the argument further. On her account, the male domination of women, or *patriarchy*, is everywhere expressed through the systematic destruction or mutilation of women. Different cultures do this in different ways: suttee (the burning alive of widows) in India; foot-binding in China; female circumcision in Muslim Africa; the burning of witches in Europe; and gynaecological therapies such as hysterectomy in modern America — *'gynocide'* as she terms it.

> Widows in that country [India] have been described as 'choosing' to be consumed by fire, when in reality Indian society makes life untenable for women left alone. Similarly American women show signs of 'willingness' to be consumed, in this case by gynaecological 'treatment'. The doctors claim that women 'ask' for it ... what is not mentioned is the fact that the patriarchs of this society also attempt to reduce women's potential for long and full living to (at best) merely not dying. (Daly, 1979, p.260)

This is a powerful argument, but it depends for its full force on whether hysterectomy seriously reduces 'women's potential for long and full living'. And here some disturbing psychological evidence has been gathered.

The psychological effects of hysterectomy

The letter to *Good Housekeeping* cited earlier commented 'now, after 11 months I have been seeing a psychiatrist for the last two for severe depression, which not only affects me but my whole family.'

☐ Why might hysterectomy have these psychological consequences?

■ Three sorts of arguments have been produced. First, the womb may perhaps have some physiological functions which directly affect mental state. Second, it might also represent the very core of womanhood to all or many women. Those women who value their maternal qualities might see these as being destroyed. Finally, what is the effect of this operation on a woman's sexual pleasure?

Some male surgeons are clearly insensitive to these psychological consequences. Here, for example, is a quotation from another letter to *Good Housekeeping*: 'Have seen how ill and debilitated my mother became after severe haemorrhaging, I am glad that I did not have to wait so long but I still half regret having had this "unnecessary piece of plumbing" (a Registrar's pre-op description) removed'. (Rivaz, 1982, p.40) Likewise, many women are offended by medical slang for the uterus — the 'box' or the 'nursery' (as opposed to the 'play-pen' for the vagina.)

Not all doctors, have, however, been so insensitive. Medical worries about the possible psychiatric consequences of hysterectomy seem to have begun in the United States in the early 1940s, shortly before Norman Miller's attack on the necessity of operating on quite so many women. Over the years, a large body of psychiatric research has been undertaken in the United States and in Britain, the great majority of which has found clinical depression in many women who have undergone hysterectomy. A review of the research in 1977 concluded that of twenty-one serious studies, fifteen had found there to be serious adverse psychological reactions. Moreover, those studies which compared such effects with those experienced by women undergoing other major operations such as cholecystectomy (the removal of the gall-bladder) had found the effects of hysterectomy to be considerably worse. On this evidence, the Daly thesis about gynocide might well be right.

Despite this evidence, and despite the fervour and variety of its critics, hysterectomy has continued to be performed on a massive scale. During the last decade, the American rate has continued to rise, even if more slowly.*

☐ Why might this be so?

■ The opponents of hysterectomy will point to the power of the medical profession, particularly surgeons, and to its continued dominance by men. However, if you are a supporter of hysterectomy, you may have argued that many of the conditions which it is used to treat are a very great burden to women. You may also have questioned whether all women see the womb as central to their womanhood.

---

* The British rate has stayed at the same level except in Scotland, where it has risen quite sharply.

In fact, women themselves disagree on the issue; just as there are fervent female opponents of hysterectomy, so there are equally fervent supporters. The article in *Good Housekeeping* that was so critical of the operation and produced the two letters cited earlier was itself attacked by some women. Here are two examples:

> Rubbish! The article made me furious. My hysterectomy was the best thing that ever happened to me. I've never been healthier in my life. My "femininity" is not centred between my legs. I feel more feminine *not* worrying about if I'll bleed or spot through my white skirt. I have no scars and couldn't recommend the operation enough. (Wilmoth, 1982, p.39)

> I am 50 years old and have had a hysterectomy within the last four years. After the first 48 hours I never looked back. I wished I had had the operation done over 20 years previously which would have given me and my family far less worries about me and my particular problems. (Rawlings, 1982, p.39)

Hysterectomy clearly needs yet further examination.

A great impediment to women

As we saw earlier the doctors and pharmacists who wrote *Diseases and Remedies* in 1898 thought that 'the menstrual periods' were a great impediment to a woman, even 'under the best of circumstances'. How great a burden are they? Tables 7.1 and 7.2 give the results from two British surveys of women's ordinary menstrual experience. Study the tables carefully and then answer the question which follows.

☐ How serious an impediment is menstruation to women's ordinary lives?

■ It appears to be quite serious for a fairly large number of women: 6 per cent report severe tension, depression or anxiety: more than 10 per cent report severe pain, headaches and irritability during menstruation;

Table 7.2 Subjective experience of menstruation in 266 women in two east Oxford practices

Subjective experience	Percentage of sample
periods longer than 5 days	33
clots	53
more than 20 pads/tampons	32
flooding	27
heavy periods, interfering with activities (in last 6 months)	26

(Gath *et al.*, 1984)

and around 30 per cent experience a moderate degree of pain, periods that last more than five days at a time, having to use a large number of pads or tampons, and flooding and general interference with ordinary activities.

There are, of course, some problems with these data. The reports are subjective, so what one woman regards as severe another may describe as moderate or even trivial. Second, the tables do not tell us how far individual women experienced some or all of these problems. Third, the questions cover only problematic aspects of menstruation. Some women may positively enjoy their monthly periods, even though they also experience pain; to them such bleeding may represent the core of their womanhood. Finally, both studies were designed and conducted primarily by doctors; women themselves might have framed the questions differently.

So menstruation may not be a great impediment to every woman. Nonetheless, the evidence so far does suggest that many women do experience it as such. Despite this, not all doctors seem to take these problems seriously. Indeed, one psychiatric interpretation has held that women with severe pain are 'characterized by a deep resentment of their feminine role'. And one gynaecology textbook, after a description of menstrual pain goes on to suggest that '... very little can be done for the patient who prefers to use

Table 7.1 Prevalence and severity of menstrual symptoms in a randomly selected group of 500 British women aged 18 to 45

Symptom	Number of women	Percentage suffering symptom to	
		moderate degree	severe degree
pain	463	32.8	12.3
headache	459	10.5	11.3
irritability	463	20.9	11.4
depression/anxiety/tension/nervousness	459	17.2	6.1
swelling	457	71.8% reported some swelling	

(Kessel and Coppen, 1963, p.62)

menstrual symptoms as a monthly refuge from responsibility and effort'. Of course, some women may well do this. As we saw in our discussion of the sick role in Chapter 3, all of us can use pain and disease as a refuge from our responsibilities on occasion. However, recent research has suggested that menstrual pain is induced by biochemical changes in the uterus. Moreover, not all gynaecologists take menstrual disorders so lightly. Indeed, the widespread prevalence of these disorders is one of the key arguments of those who advocate that hysterectomy should be used on a wide scale.

There are also other grounds for advocating hysterectomy. When it was first introduced there were few, if any, alternative treatments that offered serious relief. Nowadays, there are many treatments but, even so, all of them have their drawbacks. 'Dilatation and curettage', which involves scraping the walls of the womb under anaesthetic, is now the commonest operation in Britain, but there is little evidence that it offers much systematic relief. One study has claimed that '40 per cent of patients report improvement'; another said that such improvements were 'incidental only'; and a third, which actually measured the amount of blood lost during menstruation before and after the operation, found that bleeding was reduced for the first period after the operation but not at all thereafter (Vessey et al., 1979). Other treatments are more effective but are also more dangerous. In the 1940s radium therapy was the treatment of choice for menorrhagia. It has long since been discontinued. Hormone therapy for menstrual problems has become increasingly popular but it, too, in a minority of women, can have most undesirable effects. There is, in other words, no treatment for menstrual complaints which is simple, effective and free from complications.

Hysterectomy may have its drawbacks, but these must be weighed against the costs that other modes of treatment involve. Moreover, recent research suggests that some of the costs of hysterectomy may be less than has hitherto been thought.

Some women claim that hysterectomy has had a terrible psychological effect on them, others that they have never felt better. Whom should we believe? Perhaps both claims are true. Until very recently, it was hard to tell for, although there had been quite a large amount of research, it had all been conducted *after* women had had the operation.

☐　If we want to estimate the effects of hysterectomy on women's mental condition, what is the drawback of doing research only *after* they have had the operation?
■　We can have no idea of what it was like beforehand. If women's mental state before hysterectomy is worse before the operation than after it, then the operation is a success rather than a disaster.

At the time of writing (1984), three studies, two British and one American, had monitored the mental state of women both before and after hysterectomy. In all three of these *prospective* or longitudinal studies, women's mental state was, by and large, better after the operation than it was beforehand. The largest and best controlled of these studies was conducted by a British psychiatrist, Dennis Gath, and his colleagues. They limited their study to 156 women who were undergoing hysterectomy for menorrhagia and they interviewed the women in their homes a month before the operation, a month after, and finally eighteen months afterwards. Some of their results are given in Table 7.3. Study the table and then answer the question overleaf.

Table 7.3 Frequency of psychiatric problems in a general population sample of women and in a group of patients undergoing hysterectomy for menorrhagia

	Percentage reporting the syndrome		
Problem	General population (237 women)	1 month before hysterectomy (156 women)	18 months after hysterectomy (148 women)
worry	45	89	61
physical features of depression	9	85	37
tension	33	77	64
irritability	17	62	22
situational anxiety	28	55	48
lack of energy	8	53	27
simple depression	16	47	24
social unease	23	43	28
general anxiety	6	40	22
loss of interest and concentration	12	31	20

(Gath *et al.*, 1982, p.340)

☐ What do you think is the effect on women's mental state of (a) menorrhagia, and (b) hysterectomy?

■ The data confirm the view of the authors of *Diseases and Remedies* — that with menorrhagia a woman's 'life may become a burden to her'. The data also suggest that hysterectomy may go some way towards alleviating this burden, even though after eighteen months these women still have more psychiatric problems than the general population.

This research also looked at the sexual experience of women before and after hysterectomy. Six months after the operation, 17 per cent reported that sex was worse, 41 per cent thought it was unchanged and 39 per cent thought it had improved. As for frequency, 56 per cent reported that they now had sex more often. Finally, some attempt was made to ask women about their feelings of 'femininity': a large majority reported them as undiminished after the operation. In summary, whereas the operation may have affected some women badly, it appears to have been psychologically beneficial in the majority of cases.

The feminist critique revisited

Not all feminists have gone along with every part of the attack on hysterectomy. Moreover, we have already seen that both sides in the dispute over the operation can claim to be acting on behalf of women. Take first the selling of the operation. Many gynaecologists seem to feel that it is women who are putting the pressure on them, not the other way around. An editorial in the *British Medical Journal* states:

> Many women today regard hysterectomy as a matter for their decision rather than the doctor's. While all surgery should be approached in the light of the patient's wishes, it is a fine but crucial distinction for the doctor between making the patient an informed partner in the decision and abrogating responsibility, merely extirpating her uterus on demand. (*British Medical Journal*, 1977, p.715)

Whom should we believe? At present, the balance must lie with the feminist critics. There is by now quite a large body of research into medical consultation. Its conclusions are fairly unanimous — doctors, not patients, normally wield most power. Doctors have plenty of practice in selling their ideas, patients do not. Surgeons are liable to seem passive victims only to one another. However, the shift in attitude towards hysterectomy over the last 100 years that is manifest in the huge growth of the rate of operation must have involved changes in perception for both surgeons and for women. Many women now probably do expect to have a hysterectomy: their mother may have had one, and so

may their sister. Why should not they, if they so wish it? It seems most unlikely that many women actually 'demand' of a surgeon that he 'extirpate their uterus'. Nevertheless, just as some surgeons undoubtedly pressure unwilling women into hysterectomy, so, at least occasionally, the reverse may occur, even in a health system like the National Health Service. Now let us turn to the more radical argument that hysterectomy itself is merely the latest example of age-old masculine brutality.

☐ What evidence for and against this has been cited so far?

■ Some gynaecological motivation, both past and present, looks a little dubious. And there is evidence of appalling masculine brutality towards women in British and many other cultures. Whether this applies to hysterectomy is less certain. Quite large numbers of women complain of menstrual disorders, and hysterectomy appears to remove, or at least to diminish, some of their most serious physical and mental consequences. Even if we accept the argument that some surgeons are sadists, it would appear that they may still have been helping women at the same time as gratifying themselves.

Other evidence can also be cited against the more radical position. Mary Daly's argument relies on the fact that only women can undergo hysterectomy, and that rates of hysterectomy are extremely high: 1 in 5 British women undergo the operation. But there are other operations, also in the genital area, which only men undergo or which are performed mainly on men and which also occur at very high rates. Table 7.4 compares the rates of hysterectomy with those of prostatectomy and hernia repair. Hysterectomy is thus not the only high-volume operation. Nor do all high-volume operations or all high-volume operations in a sensitive area concern women. Moreover, how would the Daly thesis explain the large difference between the British and America hysterectomy rates? Is American culture more 'gynocidal', or is hostility to women expressed in a different form in Britain, or do we need to move to another level of analysis to explain these differences?

Table 7.4 Number of operations per 100 000 population for three common operations in England and Wales in 1975

	Males	Females
hysterectomy	—	228
prostatectomy	106	—
hernia	209	22

(data from McPherson *et al.*, 1981, p.276)

National differences in surgical decision-making

Let us begin by considering some international variations in surgical rates. Table 7.5 presents the rates by gender for three operations in England and Wales, Canada and the United States.

Table 7.5 Numbers of operations per 100 000 population for three common operations in England and Wales, Canada, and the United States in 1975

	England and Wales		Canada		United States	
	M	F	M	F	M	F
hysterectomy	—	228	—	572	—	670
prostatectomy	106	—	231	—	263	—
hernia	209	22	419	52	480	60

(data from McPherson *et al.*, 1981, p.276)

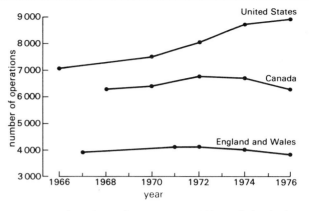

Figure 7.4 The volume of surgery per 100 000 population in the United States, Canada, England and Wales. (Vayda *et al.* 1982, p.847)

☐ Study Table 7.5 carefully. Can you detect any consistent national differences in the rates of operation?
■ For each of the three operations, England and Wales have the lowest rate, Canada is next, and the United States has the highest.

In other words, there seems to be a distinctive '*national' level of surgery*, which is relatively independent of any particular operation. This impression is confirmed, if we now examine Figure 7.4, which shows the total number of operations of all types performed in these countries over a decade. We noted earlier that the number of hysterectomies performed has continued to rise in the United States, despite some attempts to reduce it. In England and Wales, the rate, however, stayed more or less constant. Examine Figure 7.4 and then answer the following question.

☐ What happened to other operations during this period in the United States and in England and Wales? How does this compare with what has happened to hysterectomy?
■ In both cases, the changes or otherwise in the hysterectomy rate seem to have merely reflected much broader trends in an overall national rate of surgery.

What might explain these national differences? There are three main sorts of answer. One that is often favoured by surgeons is that the amount of disease differs between countries and this is reflected in the volume of operations. The second is that differences in each country's economic and social organisation produce a distinctive national volume of surgery — how wealthy the country is; the way it organises its health services; the kind of doctors it has, and so on. And the third is that there are distinct national traditions in health beliefs and theories of disease.

Studies in other areas, for example cancer, suggest that the *incidence of disease* does vary considerably between countries. So this might account for the variation in surgical rates. Unfortunately, however, in the case of hysterectomy, the only measure we have for the amount of surgically related disease in these countries is the surgical rates themselves! There is little or no independent evidence available to study the relationship of one to the other. All we can do, therefore, is see how plausible the relationship looks, and whether there are other possibly more powerful explanations. One argument against a purely disease-based explanation is that it seems unlikely that disease will vary quite so systematically between countries so closely related.

Let us, therefore, now consider some social and economic factors which seem to have a major impact on the rate of surgery. As before, we shall explore this through hysterectomy. These factors are the internal structure of the medical profession, in particular the degree of *monopoly power* enjoyed by gynaecologists; the method of health service organisation, in particular the method of medical payment; and finally, the level of *national income*. This last factor seems to bear a close relationship to the volume of all types of medical and surgical intervention.

Take monopoly power first. The British and American medical professions have had a very different history. When anaesthetics and antisepsis enabled the development of modern surgical techniques in the late nineteenth century, there was a huge surgical boom in the United States. People in other areas rushed into surgery. From that time onwards, Americans have seen surgery as a solution to many problems that are treated differently in Britain. For there was no equivalent boom in the United Kingdom. In nineteenth-century United States, specialists had failed to get a legal monopoly on certain sorts of medical practice, so there was no way that they could exclude the newcomers. But in Britain such monopolies dated back to the sixteenth century and were tightened up dramatically when the new opportunities for surgery appeared. The number of British surgeons stayed relatively small and has remained so to the present day (see Figure 7.5).

In consequence, although each British surgeon operates a lot more frequently than most American practitioners, the restriction in their numbers seems likely to have played an important part in keeping the overall volume of surgery at a lower level. But this is not the only plausible explanation. There is also the difference in the way people are paid for providing medical care and the very considerable difference in national income.

□ Norman Miller, the Chicago gynaecologist, had a theory about the possible effect of the method of payment upon the volume of hysterectomy. What was it?

■ He talked about the 'remunerative or hip-pocket hysterectomy'; in other words, he claimed that, where they had a financial incentive, surgeons would operate rather more than they would otherwise.

Financial incentives can work in different ways. As we saw earlier, in some traditional societies, the healer was paid only when, and if, the patient got better. In industrialised societies, the doctor or the surgeon is paid irrespective of whether they cure the patient. However, there are two distinct systems for making this payment. The first of these is the direct payment or piece-rate system — the surgeon who performs the hysterectomy is paid for that particular operation. The payment may be made by the patient, a relative, an employer, an insurance company, or the State, but it is always for the specific operation. In the other system, however, surgeons get a fixed salary, irrespective of the number of operations they perform.

□ Which system is more likely to provide surgeons with a financial incentive to perform hysterectomies?

■ The direct payment system, commonly known as the 'private' or 'fee-for-service' system.

Very few countries publish comparable national statistics of surgery. However, both Britain and Norway, where most surgeons are salaried, have similar 'low' rates, both for surgery in general and for hysterectomy, whereas the United States and Canada, where surgery is mostly 'fee-for-service' (piece-rate) have much higher rates. The trend in the Canadian surgery rates shown in Figure 7.3 is further interesting evidence: as the figure shows, the rate was rising until around 1972, when it started to decline. This change coincided with changes in the way that Canadian health care was funded and surgeons financed, reducing their incentive to undertake surgery. So the method of payment clearly exerts an important influence. So also might the level of national wealth. The United States is twice as rich

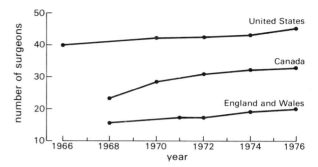

Figure 7.5 The number of surgeons per 100 000 population in the United States, Canada, England and Wales 1966–76. (Vayda *et al.* 1982, p.851)

per head of the population as Britain. It also does twice as much surgery. Perhaps the two are connected? There is quite a lot of evidence that the volume of medical treatment in industrialised countries may be in some way related to national wealth.

Conclusions

Let us close this discussion of the rights and wrongs of hysterectomy with two further comments. It may help to summarise the argument so far. It has been a fairly complex argument because every medical treatment is shaped by a great range of biological and social factors. To understand hysterectomy, we have had to look at the following: the history of the operation and the historical origins of the debate over its widespread use; the internal disputes between surgeons and the different views of different women; the various menstrual and uterine disorders for which the operation is performed and their frequency in the general population; the evidence concerning the possible prophylactic effects of hysterectomy, and its various physical and mental side-effects; the range of alternative treatments and their pros and cons; and finally, the various social and economic factors which also seem to influence the rate at which it is performed — gender relationships, the method by which surgeons are paid, the degree of professional monopoly and the level of national income.

Now consider these matters from two further perspectives. First, note that in viewing hysterectomy, it is possible to go yet wider still. For, although we have looked at both international and historical evidence we have stayed fairly close to the present day and to familiar societies. To get a wide-angle view, we need to consider what anthropologists have to say. It may also help to speculate a little about the distant future.

Menstruation can be a great impediment to a woman. Has it always been quite such a burden? Studies of non-literate peoples in traditional societies have suggested that, for many women, menstruation is considerably less frequent than in industrialised societies. Menstruation ceases during pregnancy, and in such societies, most women have large numbers of children. Prolonged suckling, which is the standard method of feeding young babies, also seems to prevent menstruation. A baby suckling at its mother's breast activates a hormone which both promotes milk secretion and delays menstruation. Moreover, regular monthly menstruation, even in a non-pregnant and non-breastfeeding woman, occurs only with adequate nutrition. Where diet is poor, limited or irregular, amenorrhoea is frequent, monthly menstruation might be the exception rather than the rule. Thus, contemporary women's experience of menstruation may be rather different from that of their predecessors. Some of the key problems which hysterectomy is used to treat may have been less of a problem in the past.

Now let us turn to the future. Begin by reconsidering one of the letters from *Good Housekeeping*: 'My "femininity" is not centred between my legs. I feel more feminine *not* worrying about if I'll bleed or spot through my white skirt.' For some women and some surgeons, there is nothing sacred about the uterus. It is a purely disposable part of the body, something to be got rid of at one's personal convenience. One famous British gynaecologist used to remark that women should be born with zippers across the abdomen, so that the womb could be thrown away more easily. Such comments may strike many people as callous, even immoral. One thing to note about them, however, is that they are relatively new. As we have seen, it was only around the turn of this century that surgery became sufficiently safe for it to be used on a wide scale. Until that time, and barring accidents, people had to put up with the particular limbs, organs and shape that they were born with. These items could not be removed or re-modelled with any ease. So the development of modern surgery has offered many possibilities that did not exist before. On one interpretation, the more dubiously motivated surgeons have used this opportunity to fool the public into submitting to unnecessary, even harmful procedures. On this account, such exploitation will disappear once both health services and the wider society are properly organised.

But there are other possibilities and interpretations. On the previous account, the individual body is sacred and surgical modification of the body can be justified only where there is serious evidence of disease. This is not the only point of view. Not everyone likes their body. As the technical capacity of surgery develops, the more people may use it to modify the bits they do not like and to remove the parts they no longer want. From this perspective, high rates of hysterectomy may be seen as part of a much broader type of surgical innovation, which also includes cosmetic surgery and the delivery of babies through Caesarean operation in order to preserve the mother's figure.

This particular use of surgery is usually frowned on by the National Health Service and by insurance companies. However, where individual patients have the money, such procedures are now quite common. In Brazil, most upper-class women now seem to give birth through a Caesarean operation and many have their faces, breasts, stomachs and thighs surgically modified as they grow older. Such cosmetic surgery is increasingly sought by men also. How this may develop in future, whether it will spread to other classes in society, cannot be foreseen with any accuracy. It should be remembered, however, that the detailed re-wiring and re-sculpting of the human body is only 100 years old. Other major changes may well lie in store.

Now let us go back over the argument so far and reconsider a theme which runs throughout most of the conventional literature. Much of the debate about hysterectomy has been dominated by an *individual model of decision-making*. We have considered what gynaecologists might choose when faced with different signs and symptoms. We have contrasted this with what women themselves might want. But individual choice does not operate in a vacuum: if Indian widows do not 'choose' to be burnt, how far do gynaecologists 'choose' to operate with one set of criteria rather than another? The choices that all of us make are constrained by the wider world of which we are a part. However, the 'medical model', the classical textbook approach in medicine, is oriented towards the individual doctor and the individual patient. The classic patient's critique of medicine is, likewise, individually focused; it is based, as are the letters to *Good Housekeeping*, on individual experience. Both these versions operate in an ideal world; a purely medical world where the only issues are clinical; an ideal patient's world where the only considerations are personal. But as we have seen in this chapter, sexual, social, economic and political relationships also have a major role in the determination of hysterectomy.

Objectives for Chapter 7

When you have studied this chapter, you should be able to:

7.1 Describe the history both of hysterectomy and of the debate over its widespread use.

7.2 Compare and contrast the key points made by the various critics of hysterectomy and those who defend it.

7.3 Describe the way in which medical decision-making is shaped, not just by individual choices, but by wider social forces.

Questions for Chapter 7

1 *(Objective 7.1)* 'Anaesthesia came quickly into use and slower and more careful operations became possible. But the range and volume of surgery remained extremely limited. Infections took a heavy toll in all "capital" operations, as major surgery was so justly called . . . very rarely did the surgeon penetrate the major bodily cavities and then only in desperation when every other hope had been exhausted.' (Starr, 1982, p.156)

(a) Of what period was this written?

(b) When did major surgery such as hysterectomy begin to be practised on a wider scale?

2 *(Objective 7.2)* '[In America] the signs are that hysterectomy is increasingly being chosen by women who are well-informed and who can afford it, as an investment against cancer, pregnancy, menstruation and menopausal disturbance of uterine function.' (*The Lancet*, 1977, p.232)

Evaluate this judgement from the perspectives of the critics of hysterectomy.

3 *(Objective 7.2)* 'There were an estimated 2.4 million unnecessary surgeries performed in 1974 at a cost to the American public of almost $4 billion. These unnecessary surgeries led to 11,900 unnecessary deaths.' This is the conclusion of the American Congressional Report on Unnecessary Surgery (1974), a report which covered every type of operation. Remembering the arguments for and against hysterectomy, what criticism would you make of this statement?

4 *(Objective 7.3)* 'In Britain, the Health Service rather than the patient is responsible for rationing and the broad selection of who shall have what . . . . While many doctors feel that such decisions increasingly are pre-empted by Government policy in allocating resources, the final allocation still rests with the clinician who must make two distinct judgements — on the net benefit to each patient and on the opportunity costs of using his (or her) own limited resources to treat one type of problem rather than another ... however highly the British Health Service patient may judge the benefit to herself of elective hysterectomy, her chances of obtaining it are small when she has to compete with more demonstrably ill patients.' (*The Lancet*, 1977, p.232)

(a) What three factors are mentioned here as potentially determining the rate of hysterectomy?

(b) What is and should be the order of their importance, according to the author of the editorial?

(c) What other factors might influence the British rate of hysterectomy?

8

Hysteria:
a diagnostic
epidemic?

During this chapter you will need the Course Reader for the article 'The hysterical woman: sex roles and role conflict in 19th-century America' by Carroll Smith-Rosenberg (Part 1, Section 1.4).

The factors which generate a particular rate of hysterectomy are complex and controversial. Nevertheless, there are several areas in which there is now solid evidence and there will be more to come in the future. It is hard to have quite the same confidence in the debates over hysteria. After 2 500 years there is no agreement even over its existence. Some deny it; others assert that it is surprisingly common.

Let us plunge straight in by examining the most famous of all cases of hysteria, that of 'Anna O', a patient treated by a Viennese doctor, Josef Breuer, from 1880 to 1882. Bertha Pappenheim, to give her her real name, eventually recovered and went on to become a leading German feminist. Her fame in medical history rests on the method of treatment which she and Breuer jointly created, the method which Sigmund Freud, then an associate of Breuer's, later developed into psychoanalysis. Our interest, however, lies in the classic description of a nineteenth-century form of hysteria which the case-notes on her sufferings provide (Sulloway, 1980 pp.54–9).

At the time that Breuer first saw her, Bertha Pappenheim was 21 years old, had been nursing her dying father for several months and was in a state of complete mental and physical exhaustion. Her symptoms were severe and extensive: rigid paralysis and loss of sensation on the right side of her body; similar but more occasional paralysis on the left side; severely disturbed eye movements and power of vision; sporadic deafness; a peculiar head posture; a repeated cough; an aversion to most food and drink (at one stage she lived for several weeks upon oranges); suicidal impulses; sporadic loss of the capacity to speak German (though her command of English remained perfect); and daily bouts of delirium, followed by a trance state. An extraordinary range of symptoms, made even more puzzling by the fact that there appeared to be no organic disease, no underlying physical condition which was causing them. Fortunately, and unlike many such patients,

Bertha Pappenheim eventually recovered — how far Breuer's therapy was responsible is unclear. Even more puzzling is the fact that this form of hysteria itself seems to have vanished. To nineteenth-century doctors, hysteria was one of the most famous and most baffling of all medical conditions; according to many .doctors, it has now disappeared in this country, though it is still common in others. An editorial in the *British Medical Journal* commented 'Hysteria (virtually a historical curiosity in Britain) is still the most common form of neurosis seen in psychiatric hospitals in India.' (1976, p.601). Such historial and international fluctuations in its incidence suggest that hysteria too might be viewed as an epidemic disease. What are its causes; has it any modern Western equivalents? And what might it tell us about the medical and social relationships between men and women? These are the questions we shall address in this and the next chapter.

Mass hysteria

Anna O's condition disappeared. But hysteria seems to take several different forms. Here, for instance, is a modern report of a possible example of 'mass hysteria':

> On Sunday 13 July, 280 children at a jazz band contest held near Mansfield collapsed in rapid succession and were taken to hospital. Most of them recovered rapidly, though seven were kept in hospital overnight. The hospital described the symptoms as

being consistent with reactions to fumes, and subsequently many other explanations were proposed. These ranged from high frequency radio waves to mass hysteria.

A striking feature was the the speed with which everything happened. An eye-witness said that she "had never seen anything like it — some of the kids were catching their friends as they fell, and then they were falling themselves. No one could understand what was happening. It looked just like a battlefield with bodies everywhere." Other symptoms that appeared were: shaking, nausea, vomiting, running eyes, sore throats, and a metallic taste in the mouth.

Extra nurses and off-duty policemen were brought in, and investigations were begun by environmental health officers, an agricultural inspector and an official from the Forestry Commission. Food poisoning was initially incriminated, and an ice-cream salesman was mobbed by angry parents. The epidemic attracted prominent coverage on television, became front-page news, and prompted the writing of this article.

The cause of the outbreak is not certain, but from descriptions of similar occurrences in the past, it is unlikely that a physical cause will be found. It will probably come to be seen as yet another manifestation of mass hysteria. (Ashton and Edwards, 1980, p.166)

Table 8.1 Some recent possible cases of mass hysteria

Case 1 Television assembly plant in Singapore	
Number affected	84 females in workforce of 802 (90 per cent female)
Symptoms	Screaming, fainting, fear, anxiety, trance states, violent acts
Trigger	No clear trigger; spirit possession reported as cause
Investigator's observations	Outbreak involved only Malay females. Hysteria spread to two neighbouring plants and lasted about two weeks. Tranquillisers did not alleviate symptoms. Medicine man called in to exorcise spirits but did not prevent additional outbreaks
Case 2 Manufacturing plant in south-eastern United States	
Number affected	89 females, 59 males in workforce of 290
Symptoms	Dizziness, nausea, difficulty breathing, bad taste in mouth, headaches
Trigger	Strange odour
Investigator's observations	Work was perceived as monotonous and boring with high production pressure
Case 3 London teaching hospital (the Royal Free)	
Number affected	102 female nurses
Symptoms	Malaise, headaches, nausea, dizziness, palpitations
Trigger	Some suggest an outbreak of 'benign myalgic encephalitis' (believed to be caused by a virus, as yet unidentified)
Investigator's observations	Those affected had more hospital admissions and more sick days from work than those who were not. Likewise, they were classified as more neurotic on the Eysenck personality test

(data taken from Colligan and Murphy, 1982, pp.33–52)

Hysteria is a commonly used word, but, in the cases of Anna O and of the Mansfield children, it is being used in a technical medical sense. In this special sense, hysteria refers to a condition in which the sufferer exhibits major physical symptoms of disease without there being any apparent physical cause. It is therefore classified as a *mental* condition which mimics organic disease.

☐ What are the main differences between the cases of Anna O and the Mansfield children?

■ Anna O was a single case whereas in Mansfield 280 children were affected almost simultaneously. Moreover, whereas the children's symptoms were relatively mild and they soon made a rapid recovery, Anna O's were extremely severe and took years to disappear.

If the kinds of symptoms that Anna O suffered are rare, 'mass hysteria' is still quite frequently reported. Table 8.1 gives summaries of three fairly recent cases reported from factories and other places of work in Britain, Singapore and the United States.

☐ The three cases cited in Table 8.1 are a cross-section of twenty-three cases reviewed in Colligan and Murphy's study. What factors do they suggest might be important in generating mass hysteria? What else do they suggest about this condition?

■ First, that most, though not all, of the sufferers seem to be women; second, that the work is sometimes described as boring and repetitive; third, that the British and American complaints are less extreme than those of the Malaysian workers and resemble those of the Mansfield children; fourth, note how the Singapore plant used both Western and traditional medicine to combat the problem: fifth, that certain sorts of personality may be particularly prone; and sixth, that those affected may also be more prone to report sick in other circumstances.

Such findings are interesting, though often disputed. Now let us turn to some evidence that individual hysteria may still be with us, though usually, it would seem, in a less dramatic form than that exhibited by Anna O.

Briquet's Syndrome

Paul Briquet was a French doctor who in 1859 published his *Treatise on Hysteria*, a study based on detailed clinical investigation of 430 cases seen at the Hôpital de la Charité in Paris, cases whom he compared with 167 sick but non-hysterical patients. Briquet was only one of many well-known doctors who published on the topic. He has been famous for two things: first, for his pioneering use of statistics in psychiatry and, second, for his systematic critique of the traditional theory of hysteria which stressed the role of the uterus. In the 1940s, his work was revived by

a group of American psychiatrists centred around James J. Purtell of St Louis. These modern researchers have defined an extreme form of the condition which they call Briquet's Syndrome, since the term is less pejorative than hysteria. On their definition, the syndrome is a chronic illness occurring almost entirely in women and beginning before the age of 30. Women with this condition have a dramatic, vague or complicated medical history and a large number of unexplained symptoms. To qualify for the syndrome

the symptom must have led the patient to see a physician, caused her to take medicine other than aspirin, or it must have interfered substantially with the patient's life . . . . (Woodruff *et al.*, 1971, p.426)

the patient must report at least 25 medically unexplained symptoms for a diagnosis . . . in at least nine out of ten symptom groups [see Table 8.2, overleaf] and 20 to 24 symptoms for a "probable" diagnosis. (Kroll *et al.*, 1979, p.171)

☐ Why might Purtell *et al.* have insisted on having twenty-five symptoms for a diagnosis, rather than just one or two?

■ They deemed it wise to make the diagnosis as rigorous as possible, for two main reasons. First, all of us get some of these symptoms from time to time without any apparent organic cause. Second, how is it possible to be absolutely sure that there is no organic illness present?

Let us consider these points further. First, everyone seems to get the occasional hysterical symptom from time to time. This in itself does not warrant a diagnosis of hysteria. Only when people regularly take a large number of such symptoms to a doctor is it appropriate to talk in these terms. Second, the danger of misdiagnosis, of defining someone as hysterical when they have, in fact, a serious organic illness, is clearly a grave problem. Thomas Willis, a seventeenth-century physician, wrote this about hysteria: 'Among the diseases of women, hysterial affection is of such bad repute ... it must bear the faults of numerous other affections ...' Putting this into more modern language, the authors of one research paper on Briquet's Syndrome note that:

The authors have seen patients with brain tumours, meningococcus meningitis, intestinal obstruction, tetanus, cancer of the oesophagus, cancer of the stomach, uterine cancer, typhoid fever, pernicious vomiting of pregnancy, chorioepithelioma, postpartum sagittal sinus thrombosis, normal pregnancy, bacterial endocarditis, polyneuritis and thyrotoxicosis who have been diagnosed as having hysteria or "neurosis" when inadequate criteria of diagnosis were used, with disastrous or near-disastrous consequences in some patients for the patient and embarrassment for the physician. (Cohen *et al.*, 1953, p.984)

So there are some good reasons for being careful with this particular diagnosis. Using Purtell's definition, researchers in this tradition claim to have produced the following findings: first, that the syndrome can be found in 2 per cent of women (though other research gives a lower estimate of 3–6 per 1 000); second, that it is found equally in women of every social class; third, that close relatives of women with the syndrome are ten times more likely to have the syndrome themselves than are women in the general population; fourth, that women with this condition are liable to receive a good deal of unnecessary and possibly dangerous treatment. This fourth finding is illustrated in Figure 8.1, which shows the location and number of major operations carried out on fifty women subsequently diagnosed as having Briquet's Syndrome compared with fifty 'normal' women.

Briquet claimed that the ratio of female to male sufferers was about 20:1; the modern researchers have held it to be even rarer among males, in fact, on their stringent criteria, almost non-existent. The question of whether men do or do not suffer from hysteria has been controversial for several hundred years and, like most of the hysteria story, still has no satisfactory resolution. Though it is not our topic here, it needs a brief consideration. Most traditional writers on the topic agreed with Briquet: hysteria was a woman's disease. Some, however, dissented. Sydenham (1624–89), the 'English Hippocrates', felt that it occurred in men also, though in a milder, more melancholic, form which he preferred to call hypochondria since men have no uterus. And from the nineteenth century onwards, there was an intense debate over the matter as psychiatrists noted that men too could suffer from hysterical paralysis; after railway accidents or on the battlefield, for example. In consequence, men may now be diagnosed by many doctors as suffering from some form of hysteria, though to a lesser degree than women. The condition in men, however, has received relatively little research.

Table 8.2 The ten symptom groups used in the diagnosis of Briquet's Syndrome*

Group 1	*Group 5*	*Group 9*
headaches	anorexia	back pain
sickly	weight loss	joint pain
	marked fluctuations in weight	extremity pain
Group 2	nausea	burning pains of sexual organs, mouth or
blindness	abdominal bloating	rectum
paralysis	food intolerances	other bodily parts
anaesthesia	diarrhoea	
aphonia	constipation	*Group 10*
fits or convulsions		nervousness
unconsciousness	*Group 6*	fears
amnesia	abdominal pain	depressed feelings
deafness	vomiting	need to quit working or inability to
hallucinations		carry on regular duties because of
urinary retention	*Group 7*	feeling sick
trouble walking	dysmenorrhoea	crying easily
other conversion symptoms	menstrual irregularity	feeling life was hopeless
	amenorrhoea	thinking a good deal about dying
Group 3	excessive bleeding	wanting to die
fatigue		thinking of suicide
lump in throat	*Group 8*	suicide attempts
fainting spells	sexual indifference	
visual blurring	frigidity	
weakness	dyspareunia	
dysuria	other sexual difficulties	
	vomiting during 9 months of pregnancy	
Group 4	or hospitalised for hyperemesis	
breathing difficulty	gravidarum	
palpitation		
anxiety attacks		
chest pain		
dizziness		

(Kroll *et al.*, 1979, p.172)

* Some of these terms will be unfamiliar; their precise meanings are not essential to the present argument.

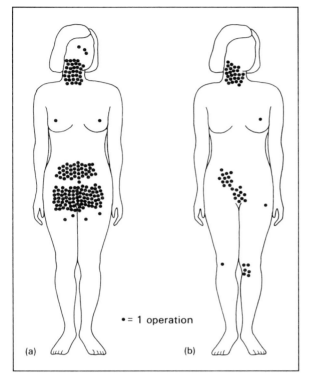

Figure 8.1 Major operations in 50 hysteria patients and 50 healthy controls. (Cohen *et al.* 1953, p.979)

• = 1 operation

(a)   (b)

Table 8.3 Precipitating factors in hysterical patients

Precipitating factor	Percentage of cases
'marital and family afflictions' (including both ill-treatment and the loss of a husband or close relative)	25
'panic after unexpected events' (such as witnessing a death, a street battle or a fire)	14
disorders of menstruation	11
'intense moral emotions' (such as the departure of loved ones, receipt of bad news, intense disputes or anger)	11
other conflicts (such as illegitimate pregnancies and tensions with mothers-in-law)	9
pregnancy, childbirth, first menstruation, bleeding, rape, 'abuse of coitus'	7
weakness after a severe illness	5
'afflictions of the heart' (such as conflicts, unsatisfied desires, unhappy marriages)	5
worry at leaving home and moving to city	4
'chlorosis' (a disease classification which has now disappeared. Chlorosis was held to be a disease of young women, characterised by anorexia, palpitations, a greenish pallor and menstrual irregularities)	3
financial reverses	3
extreme fatigue	2
observing another person having an hysterical or epileptic attack	2

(based on Mai's 1980 summary of Briquet)

Briquet presented several possible explanations for hysteria. Given its much more frequent occurrence in the close relatives of hysterical patients, he thought there might be a hereditary link.

   □ Does this imply that hysteria has a genetic component?
   ■ Not necessarily: hysterical behaviour could be 'learned' from relatives. Either explanation is compatible with the data.

Briquet also paid close attention to the circumstances that seemed to precipitate the condition, for he maintained that hysteria was the product of a combination of factors, both personal and environmental. To investigate these, he gathered data on the 430 cases he had seen at his Paris hospital and added material from a number of hysterical patients who had been studied by other doctors, making a total of 591 patients in all. He then analysed the precipitating factors as in Table 8.3.

   □ Can you detect any problems with the categories that Briquet used to analyse his data?
   ■ The categories overlap. For example, 'marital and family afflictions' is very close to both 'other conflicts' and 'afflictions of the heart'.

   □ What proportion of cases seemed to involve the womb, however tangentially?
   ■ At most, between 20 and 30 per cent. ('Disorders of menstruation', 'pregnancy, etc', 'other conflicts' and 'chlorosis'.)

   □ What seems to be the main type of precipitating factor?
   ■ Social conflict or things going wrong with intimate relationships ('marital and family afflictions' — 25 per cent; 'intense moral emotions' — 11 per cent; other conflicts — 9 per cent; rape and 'abuse of coitus' — up to 7 per cent; 'afflictions of the heart' — 5 per cent). Overall, somewhere between 50 and 60 per cent of all cases seemed to be precipitated by intimate social disturbances.

Doubts about hysteria

Evidence such as this has suggested to many doctors and psychologists that, whatever its origin and whatever name we give it, hysteria is a powerful, disabling and distressing condition which can lead to further serious consequences. Of course, given the way it simulates other (organic*) illnesses, it can be very hard to diagnose. Nonetheless, it seems both real and medically significant. However, such claims are fiercely disputed, both within and without the medical profession. In 1965, an English psychiatrist, Elliot Slater, traced 112 patients who had earlier been diagnosed as suffering from hysteria. Roughly ten years later, 60 per cent had been found to have some organic disease, 8 per cent had been re-diagnosed as suffering either from schizophrenia or depression, and, though those who were left could possibly be classified as suffering from hysteria, they fell into two quite distinctive groups, one matching the Briquet's Syndrome definition, the second fitting an alternative version of hysteria proposed by another group of research workers. He concluded:

> No evidence has yet been offered that patients suffering from 'hysteria' are in medically significant terms anything more than a random selection. Attempts at rehabilitation of the syndrome ... lead to mutually irreconcilable formulations, each of them determined by their terms of reference. The only thing that 'hysterical' patients can be shown to have in common is that they are all patients ... like all unwarranted beliefs which still attract credence, it is dangerous. The diagnosis of 'hysteria' is a disguise for ignorance and a fertile source of clinical error. (Slater, 1965, p.1399)

In Chapter 2 of this book we saw how many traditional disease categories, such as 'scrofula', disappeared in the light of new knowledge and new disease terms took their place. We saw how hard it was to develop clear and generally acceptable diagnostic categories.

☐ Can you recall how this was eventually achieved? (Remember the contributions of Sydenham and Morgagni.)

■ More accurate diagnosis was developed in two main steps. First, physicians like Sydenham showed the importance of detailed clinical description. Then

pathologists like Morgagni demonstrated how clinical observation must be linked to the findings of post-mortem examinations.

☐ Can you think of any difficulties in applying this method to mental illness?

■ Morgagni's method works only for diseases with an organic base. However, if some diseases are purely mental or social in origin, pathologists cannot contribute to their diagnosis. (One cannot, however, be too precise on this point. Every disease, whatever its ultimate origin, has both biological and social manifestations to a greater or lesser extent.)

The modern belief in 'mental illness' is, in fact, of very recent origin, and is still heavily disputed by many psychiatrists. Until this century, what we now call mental illness was routinely taken to have an organic cause. For example, J.-M. Charcot (1825–93), professor of pathological anatomy in the University of Paris, examined many thousands of brains in an attempt to link pathology to clinical observation. However, very few such links were successfully made. As a result, although a triumphant Whig history of physical medicine can readily be written, there is no equivalent story to be told in psychiatry. Writing in the 1930s, the American historian of medicine, Richard Shryock, argued that the state of contemporary psychiatry was rather similar to that of eighteenth-century physical medicine. Many disease classifications were heavily disputed; many influential theories of mental illness, such as psychoanalysis, were monistic (they ascribed everything to a single cause) and rested on a fragmentary and ill-researched empirical base; the entire field was riven by hostile, warring camps. In the fifty years since Shryock wrote, some important progress has been made. Nonetheless, psychiatric knowledge is still far less advanced than that of organic medicine. In consequence, psychiatry has long come under heavy attack from the general public. We have already seen how some psychiatrists have serious doubts about the meaning of 'hysteria'. An equally powerful critique has been mounted by feminist writers, a critique which is increasingly accepted, at least in part, by some psychiatrists.

The feminist critique of hysteria

Slater had doubts about the validity of the diagnosis of hysteria because of the extraordinary variation in the cases to which it was applied. But there are other grounds for doubt also. Consider the following quotations from two American psychiatrists, one a man, the other a woman:

> Hysterical can be used as a pejorative label to denigrate someone whom the psychiatrist believes to be insufficiently serious. I have had the impression that susceptible young male residents may classify as a

---

* 'Organic' is a term that indicates biologically caused disease as opposed to that from psychological causes. *Experiencing and Explaining Disease* contains a more detailed discussion of these concepts. The Open University (1985) *Experiencing and Explaining Disease*, The Open University Press. (U205 *Health and Disease*, Book VI)

hysterical personality any reasonably attractive woman with whom they come into therapeutic contact. (Chodoff, 1974, p.1076)

The diagnostic indicators of hysteria are very much in keeping with the media presentation of the female sex .... I do believe that there is a danger that the hysterical personality will be reduced to the description of a particular type of feminine behaviour that has a certain effect on a male observer. (Lerner, 1974, pp.159, 162)

To Chodoff and Lerner, the diagnosis of hysteria may often have more to do with the doctors than it does with the patient. What evidence is there for this? So far, there seem to have been no systematic studies of medical decision-making in hysteria. However, other research, conducted by an American doctor, Karen Armitage, and her colleagues (1979), may still throw some light on the issue. This study examined the medical records of 52 married couples seeing nine male doctors in a white middle-class practice in San Diego in California. Five common medical complaints were chosen for comparison: back pain, headache, dizziness, chest pain and fatigue. On the basis of the records, the wives had suffered rather more from fatigue than did their husbands, but otherwise there were no significant differences between the numbers of men and women with the various complaints. There was, however, a significant difference in the *extent* to which each sex received a detailed interview and examination from their doctor (in American medical terminology, the 'work-up'). For all five conditions, the men received a considerably more extensive work-up than the women. Armitage *et al.* also found that the women visited their doctor one-and-a-half times more often than the men.

   ☐   What do these findings suggest about the way the nine male doctors viewed men's and women's complaints?
   ■   There are at least two possibilities. The first is that, since they saw the women more often, the doctors felt that they could get away with a briefer work-up. The other possibility is that they took the women's complaints less seriously; they might, perhaps, have viewed the men as more stoical, the women as more hysterical.

This tendency, if such it is, may have serious effects on women's medical history. Consider the following hypothesis: once a psychological rather than an organic diagnosis has been made and entered into a patient's medical records, this may in turn influence the doctor's interpretation of any future illnesses. Once a patient has been *labelled* in this fashion, it may be very hard for her to escape. It may also alter her behaviour. Distressed and

disorientated by her doctor's reaction, she may vehemently insist on the physical reality of her symptoms, thus further reinforcing the initial diagnosis of hysteria. Now apply this analysis to a topic considered earlier.

   ☐   What effect might male prejudice against women have on the investigation of mass outbreaks of illness in factories?
   ■   Doctors may possibly leap to the diagnosis of mass hysteria without fully investigating the physical causes, for example, a chemical leak.

One part of the feminist critique has, therefore, questioned the reality of the diagnosis of hysteria; it asks how far does it merely, or mostly, reflect male prejudice against women. The second type of feminist criticism is rather different. This version accepts that hysteria exists (though less frequently than male prejudice would have it). However, it sees hysteria as caused largely by men and by the *subordinate role* that men ascribe women. Becoming hysterically ill is one of the few ways that some women have of coping with an intolerable situation. For an example of such analysis, turn now to the Course Reader (Part 1, Section 1.4) and study the essay by Carroll Smith-Rosenberg, 'The Hysterical Woman: Sex Roles and Role Conflict in 19th-century America'.

   Smith-Rosenberg offers what one might call a power or *conflict theory of hysteria*. Hysteria, on this theory, is the refuge or revenge of the weak. As a refuge it offers merely a prison, but a prison of the patient's own making. As revenge goes, it is a most unsatisfactory form, a Doomsday weapon which destroys the patient as well as the 'enemy' — if it were otherwise, it might be chosen more often. It is also a model with close links to the earlier discussion of the sick role.

   ☐   List any connections that occur to you between Smith-Rosenberg's discussion of hysteria and Parson's analysis of the sick role. (Turn back to the appropriate section in Chapter 3 (p.26) if necessary.)
   ■   According to Parsons, people who are sick are allowed to escape from their normal social respon-sibilities. In consequence, hysterical symptoms which mimic physical illnesses also offer such an escape. But hysterical patients do not quite fit the sick role, for hysteria is a sort of parody of sickness. Doctors therefore have a difficult time with them. In the normal sick role, it is the patient's duty to try to get better. The hysterical patient may not want to. Also, it is the doctor's duty to certify that a patient is sick — but are hysterical patients sick or just malingering? Finally, it is normally the doctor's duty to help the patient; in hysteria, whose side should the doctor be on — the patient's or the relatives? And whose side is the patient

on? Are they receiving help from the doctor, or are they instead exploiting the medical profession for their own ends? (Such problems are exacerbated in private medicine, when the patient may actually have hired the doctor.) In summary, hysteria throws all the rights and obligations of the sick role into confusion; is, indeed, almost a disease of the sick role.

☐ Now compare Smith-Rosenberg's analysis with that of Briquet. In what ways is it similar; in what ways different?
■ Like Briquet, Smith-Rosenberg sees hysteria as affecting all sorts of women and stresses conflict as a major precipitating factor. They also agree that a wide variety of situations may lead to this conflict. There are, however, some differences. Smith-Rosenberg stresses above all the relationship of men to women in Victorian society. Briquet mentions matters such as 'abuse of coitus', illegitimate pregnancies and husbands' mistreatment of their wives, but does not elaborate this into a more general theory of gender relationships. Smith-Rosenberg is also particularly interested in the doctor–patient relationship, which Briquet does not treat at this level. Finally, Smith-Rosenberg uses a more intensive literary method; Briquet relies on statistics.

Smith-Rosenberg emphasises the importance of the social relationships between men and women — that is, *gender relations* — in the understanding of hysteria. By contrast, *sexual theories* seek to root the explanation of hysteria in biological differences between males and females, and, in particular, in disorders or frustration of sexual activity. Freud held a version of this theory, as did another Edwardian prophet of sexuality, the English sexual libertarian, Edward Carpenter, an ex-priest of the Church of England. Here, in his autobiography, he looks back to the Victorian age:

> I came home in the summer to Brighton to find my sisters, for the most part unmarried, wearing out their lives and their affectional capacities with nothing to do, and nothing to care for: a little music, a little painting, a walk up and down the Promenade; but the primal needs of life unspoken and unallowed .... It is curious — and interesting in its queer way — to think that almost the central figure of the drawing room in that later Victorian age ... was a young or middle-aged woman lying supine on a couch — while around her, amiably conveying or consuming tea and coffee, stood a group of quasi-artistic or intellectual men. The conversation ranged, of course, over artistic and literary topics, and the lady did her best to rise to it; but the effort probably did her no good. For the real trouble lay far away. It was of the nature of *hysteria*

> — and its meaning is best understood by considering the derivation of that word. I had two sisters — who each of them for some twenty years led that supine, and one may say tragic, life; so I had good occasion — beside what may have lain within my own experience — to understand it pretty thoroughly. Certainly the disparity of the sexes and the absolute non-recognition of sexual needs — non-recognition either in life or in thought — weighed terribly hard upon the women of that period. (Carpenter, 1916, pp.94–5)

☐ Carpenter clearly believes that sexual deprivation is an important factor in hysteria. What other possible reasons does he point to?
■ Like Smith-Rosenberg, he holds that hysteria is caused by a lack of power ('the disparity of the sexes') and the need to fulfil oneself properly in life ('wearing out their lives and affectional capacities with nothing to do and nothing to care for'). Thus he combines explanations based on sex and those based on social gender relations.

Not all sexual theorists of hysteria have shared Carpenter's libertarian approach, either to women's sexuality or to their equality. In Chapter 9 we shall focus on the history of male theorising about women, about women's sexuality and about women's apparent propensity for hysteria. Thus far, we have considered only nineteenth- and twentieth-century history; in Chapter 9 we shall trace the story back to the Greeks and beyond. Doing so will also enable us to recap many of the themes about science, the classical tradition and folk-belief that have occurred throughout this book.

Before we begin, however, several points are worth pondering on. First, although we are currently passing through a period of revolt by many women against their treatment by men, such revolts are nothing new. The battle between the sexes goes back a long way. Men might have dominated women, but they were conscious that their control was not absolute and was sometimes resented. Thus in Chaucer's *Canterbury Tales*, the Wife of Bath, a fiercely independent woman, tells the story of a knight condemned to death for rape but whose life is spared if he can answer the question, 'What thing is it that wommen most desiren?' He fails to do so and is in complete despair. Eventually he gets the answer from an old woman and tells the queen and all her ladies who had first set him the question:

> 'My liege lady, generally,' quod he,
> 'Wommen desire to have sovreintee
> As wel as over hir housbonde as hir love,
> And for to been in maistrye him above.

This is youre most desir though ye me kille.
Dooth as you list: I am here at youre wille.'
In al the court ne was ther wif ne maide
Ne widwe that contrairied that he seyde...
(Chaucer, *The Wife of Bath's Tale*, late fourteenth
century, 1037–1044; 'maistrye' = mastery)

Given the possibility and sometimes the actuality of female
revolt, men needed some kind of warrant or authority for
their continued rule, and they regularly appealed, as they
do now, to medical, biological or religious grounds.
Theories in all of these areas might serve as a justification
for male rule; thus they might owe more to *masculine
ideology* than to science or religion. Where does hysteria
come into all this? As we shall see, many of the explanations
of hysteria were closely related to male justifications of
female subordination and it is for this reason that hysteria
has attracted so much attention from feminist historians.

For, whereas some modern writers have argued that
hysteria is a product of women's domination by men,
traditional writers reversed the proposition. For them,
women were naturally inferior and the very things that
rendered them inferior also made them liable to hysteria.
Hysteria was a proof, if proof were needed, of female
weakness, of female incompetence, and even sometimes, of
female evil.

This is not to say that all men regarded women as
inferior, or that all men treated them with the same degree
of brutality that is recorded in places in the next chapter.
Although the dominant tradition saw women as rightfully
subordinate, there were important variants within this.
Moreover, not every man held this view. Montaigne,
though no feminist, held that there were few differences
between the sexes: 'I say that males and females are cast in
the same mould, and that, education and usage excepted,
the difference is not great.' (Montaigne, 1952, p.434)

Objectives for Chapter 8

When you have studied this chapter, you should be able
to:

8.1 Describe problems in the definition and diagnosis of hysteria.

8.2 Describe the power or conflict theory of hysteria
which relates its origin to women's inferior social
position in a male-dominated society.

Questions for Chapter 8

1 (*Objective 8.1*) 'To arrive at a thoroughly warranted
positive diagnosis of "functional (hysterical) paralysis"
is often for a time impossible, even to one who has a very
extensive acquaintance with nervous diseases; at the
most such a diagnosis may be regarded as more or less
probable.' (Charlton Bastian, 1893, quoted in Slater,
1965, p.1 395)

After some hesitation, Bastian, a nineteenth-century
psychiatrist, arrives at the conclusion that it is
impossible to be absolutely certain about the diagnosis
of hysteria in a particular case. Why should this be so?

2 (*Objective 8.1*) Elliot Slater, a critic of the entire
concept of hysteria, sees its 'diagnosis' as due to a
particular form of interaction between doctor and
patient. He analyses this in the following terms:

people with say a histrionic temperament [a flair
for the dramatic] naturally lend the stamp of their
personality to their symptoms, whether they are
suffering from an organic or a neurotic disorder.
All that one can say is that these modes of
behaviour seem to constitute part of a stimulus-
response system between patient and doctor.
Unwittingly, inevitably, from his very nature, the
patient applies the hystero-diagnosis stimulus;
unwittingly, inevitably, from the long process of
conditioned training through which he has gone
the doctor reacts with the hystero-diagnostic
response. (Slater, 1965, p.1 399)

How might a feminist critic of the concept of hysteria
analyse the same situation if the patient were a woman?

3 (*Objective 8.2*) What might a conflict theory of female
hysteria make of the following observation?

In my own experience I have been struck by how
often the hysterical patient's self-image is
blemished by a sense of inauthenticity. I have also
noted that their apparent submissiveness and
eagerness to please may be transmuted on the
other side of the coin into a kind of ruthless
wilfulness which is often very disconcerting,
especially in psychotherapeutic relationships.
(Chodoff, 1982, p.545)

Hysteria... the *furor uterinus*

Chapter 8 introduced the complexities of hysteria and provided a social explanation of the phenomenon; an explanation that has currently gained quite widespread acceptance, though the long struggle over the analysis of hysteria still continues. But social, even mental, explanations of this illness are a relatively new affair. For over 2 000 years its analysis was dominated by biological or supernatural explanations, by accounts that placed the cause of the condition either in women's bodies or else in their spiritually evil predisposition. The natural, biological explanation derived from the Graeco-Arab tradition of classical medical science; the supernatural account from folklore and from the Christian tradition. In some respects, each tradition opposed the other, sometimes bitterly. Yet, for most of the time, they agreed on one thing. In both accounts, women were normally portrayed as inferior, either biologically or spiritually. And the reasons for women's general inferiority were also the reasons why some of them became hysterical. This chapter surveys the 2 000 and more years of debate over the origins of hysteria. Its principal focus is on the way different explanations were often used not just to understand women but also to keep them in their place. It also serves some other purposes. This detailed account illustrates the extraordinarily far-reaching influence of the Graeco-Arab tradition; the major struggle between the natural and supernatural traditions; the long and largely unsuccessful attempt to understand mental illness in biological terms; traditional debates over human sexuality; and the inadequacies of a purely Whig approach to medical history. Some of the people who appeared as heroes earlier on are cast in a slightly different light in what follows here.

We shall begin our account, once again, with some nineteenth-century case studies of hysteria. However, whereas Breuer's work with Anna O illustrated what was to become a classic approach of the twentieth century, one of the following accounts is based on a far older explanatory tradition. The difference between these two cases illustrates the major shift in the analysis of hysteria that took place during the nineteenth century. As you read the two case studies, pay special attention to the symptoms, the causes and the treatments. The first account was given by an eminent Parisian authority on hysteria, Jean-Baptiste Louyer-Villermay (1776–1837), and published in 1844.

A young female person of twenty-one years, endowed with a good constitution and regular in her menstrual periods, who had habitually enjoyed perfect health, met a young man several times in society who succeeded in inspiring a violent passion in her. The parents of this young lady objected to the match that she so ardently desired. From that time on, a slight disturbance in her health became noticeable, and her menstrual cycle became irregular. In the space of six months she experienced several hysterical attacks with convulsive movements, the sensation of strangulation, hysterical boils, choking, tingling in the uterus, etc. Medical treatment was limited to the prescription of a few leeches to the vulva.

Shortly afterwards, this young person found a letter from her sweetheart in her parents' possession, which they refused to give to her. She was immediately seized by an attack much stronger than the preceeding ones, which was accompanied by a lethargic coma, an absolute loss of feeling and movement, and lockjaw and rigidity of the pharynx to the extent that swallowing was nearly impossible. Her regular doctor prescribed copious bleeding by means of six leeches applied behind each ear for this condition, but the symptoms in no way diminished, and three days passed without the slightest change. It was then that I was called. I found the patient unconscious and unable to respond to questions addressed to her; she appeared to be very ill and to understand nothing at all. Her face was slightly flushed and bright, her eyes fixed, her eyelids constantly closed, and her teeth clenched, and the obstruction in her swallowing remained the same. Respiration was troubled; the pulse was faint but regular and not far from its natural state. I prescribed an infusion of lime-blossom tea, an antispasmodic potion, and two blistering agents to the thighs.

The next day, the patient was in nearly the same state. She did, however, utter a few words, but they made no sense, although they did seem to relate to her attachment [for the young man]. Moreover, a general clamminess began to manifest itself. It was deemed advisable to apply a new blistering agent to the nape of the neck, and when the sweating had been completed, compresses of salty water and vinegar were applied to her head. In addition, her neck was rubbed with oil, camphor, laudanum, and ether; finally she was given injections and partial injections of camphor and asafetida [i.e. vaginal douches of antispasmodic drugs].

At the end of seven days, this young woman recovered the use of her senses, retaining only a vague memory of the crisis that she had experienced. (quoted in Hellerstein *et al.*, 1981, pp.111–2)

The second account of hysteria was given in a lecture delivered in 1866 to students of St Bartholomew's Hospital by F.C. Skey, a former president of the Royal College of Surgeons and of the Royal Medical and Chirurgical [i.e. Surgical] Society of London. Figure 9.1 illustrates an episode of hysteria in a French hospital of this period.

It is notorious that the sight of a person under a hysteric attack has a tendency to involve other hysteric persons around her. It has happened to me several times in my Hospital career to witness the contagious, or rather the imitative, form of active or paroxysmal Hysteria on a large scale. On one of these occasions, in a ward of twelve females, no less than nine young women were affected at the same time. Some were so violent as to call for the assistance of sisters, nurses, and other servants of the establishment to restrain them; and inasmuch as a person under the influence of Hysteria brings into action all the latent strength of her muscular frame, *which is greatly in excess of her apparent strength*, the services of these attendants were scarcely sufficient for the purpose — several requiring three or four strong men to prevent injury to their persons. The attack commences in the person of one girl, who may have been the subject of some trivial operation, or been brought under the immediate influence of the disease by mental emotion. No sooner is the condition of this person observed by her fellow-patients than her influence is felt throughout the ward, and the second subject may

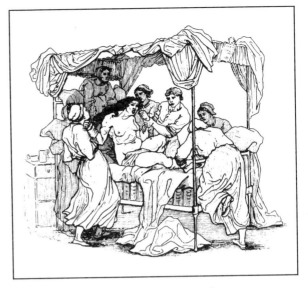

Figure 9.1 Violence des 'grands mouvements'.

become involved, occupying a bed at the remote end of the room, and thus it passes irregularly from bed to bed, each patient appearing to take the disease in the order of their constitutional liability. In the course of an hour, more or less, it subsides, and tranquillity is restored, but the evil only slumbers, and on the following day the same scene may recur — less violent, perhaps, but acted by the same persons as at first. Some of these patients, who were not affected to violence, were affected to tears and wept in silence, while some few were not implicated at all, nor did they show any tendency to sympathise with the disease.

These curious attacks, though they appear to the subjects of them irresistible, are yet but the result of what has been termed a 'surrender', and might be prevented by an adequate motive. The mode adopted to arrest this curious malady consists in bringing these persons under the influence of some powerful mental emotion, and in making some strong and sudden impression on the mind through the medium of, probably, the most potent of all impressions, fear. They are not lost to consciousness, and for the moment, except in the intensity of their paroxysm, they will listen to the voice of authority. Sympathy and kindness, or tenderness of voice and manner, are worse than useless. They rather aggravate than mitigate the evil. Ridicule, to a woman of sensitive mind, is a powerful weapon, and will achieve something; but there is no emotion equal to fear, and a threat of personal chastisement will not necessarily be required to be carried into execution. On two of the occasions I have referred to, a few quarts of cold water suddenly thrown on the person of a chief delinquent instantly brought the ward to a state of reason and subordination. The disease succumbed to the indignity of the treatment. There can be no doubt, then, that a malady spreading by sympathy and cured by fear, has its origin in the mind. (Skey, 1867, pp.61–3)

☐ In each of these cases: first, is the hysteria regarded as a *mental* or an *organic* disorder and how is the treatment apportioned to the cause? Second, what does the account reveal about the social relationships between women and men?

■ In the first account, hysteria seems to be regarded as an *organic* disorder and the cause asigned would appear to be suppressed sexual desire. The treatment focuses not only on the affected parts of the body but also on the women's erogenous zones — the vulva, ears, thighs, neck, and internal sexual organs — and, in accordance with humoral medical theory, uses leeches and counter-irritation (blistering agents).

The second account presents hysteria as a *mental* 'disease', its cause as a 'constitutional liability' beset with an 'irresistible' emotional disturbance. The treatment, therefore, consists of creating a still greater emotional *counter*-disturbance by means of ridicule, intimidation, or humiliation. Since some women 'wept in silence' while others were unable to contain themselves, it is possible to interpret these reactions as a show of emotional solidarity.

In both accounts the female patients appear to be largely passive, and men take a dominant role. It was a young man in the first account who had 'succeeded in inspiring a violent passion' in the patient. It is the male doctor's 'voice of authority' in the second account that can quell the women's attacks by 'ridicule' or 'personal chastisement'. At the same time, however, the dominance over the hysterical patient is not entirely a male role; women also play their part — the mother in the first case, the sisters and nurses in the second.

The mental theory of hysteria proposed by Skey is an example of early modern thinking in this field. Louyer-Villermay's organic account, by contrast, draws on a tradition that stretches back at least as far as the Egyptians, a tradition that is explored in the rest of this chapter. There are, however, two important points to be borne in mind. First, remember both how hard it is to define hysteria and the dangers of confusing it with other, organic conditions. Is 'mass hysteria', for example, really a relative of individual 'hysteria', and is one case the same as another? Such questions become even more difficult to answer when we study the remoter past. Was the dancing mania of the era of the Black Death a form of mass hysteria? Does the same apply to the witchcraft craze of the sixteenth and seventeenth centuries, or to the 'witches' or their supposed victims? How far did traditional medicine distinguish adequately between hysteria and epilepsy? As we saw earlier in considering plague, questions of definition create even graver problems for historical analysis than they do for contemporary research. Second, remember that there is also a patient role as well as a female role. Some of the ways in which women were treated were common to all patients, male or female. The lot of the mental patient could be hard indeed, whatever their gender. Some of the apparently brutal forms of treatment described in the next few pages were based on an early form of psychological theory and were often meted out with equal brutality to men.

Ancient afflictions

Graeco-Arab and medieval medicine inherited the Egyptian theory that the womb is like a wandering animal with an appetite for bearing children. That the womb could move was not in question: physicians had observed uterine prolapse, the partial expulsion of the womb through the vagina in difficult childbirth. This was a distressing condition, and doctors reasoned that unimpregnated women (especially those deprived of sexual relations with men) who were occasionally distressed by seizures and convulsions, also suffered from a displaced uterus, a restive, malcontented womb that had left its natural position in the pelvis and strayed upwards towards the liver, stomach, and heart. In the first century AD, the physician Aretaeus of Cappadocia noted that this 'hysteria' occurred not only in widows, but also in elderly virgins and in younger women whose wombs were generally less sedate.

The obvious prescription for hysteria of this sort was marriage. An unmarried woman was not in her natural state; her menstruation became painful and intermittent, and her womb lacked regular injections of sperm to keep it moist. So the womb dried, it became lighter, rose upwards in the body, and hysteria resulted. If the cure of marriage was impossible, physicians had recourse to fumigation: fetid smells through the mouth to repel the womb from above, fragrant smells through the vagina to lure it downward. Or like Aulus Cornelius Celsus, a medical contemporary of Aretaeus, they might try draining blood from the woman who underwent an hysterical attack, a practice that persisted for some 1 800 years.

Not all doctors believed in the theory of the *wandering womb*. In the second century AD Soranus of Ephesus and Galen of Pergamon still regarded the womb as the seat of hysteria, but did not see it as hyperactive. There was, however, still a strong sexual element in their theorising.

Soranus attributed hysteria to inflammation of the uterus. He prescribed an erotic regimen: warm compresses to the body, gentle massage, and olive oil applied to the external genitalia and adjacent regions. Galen, the foremost anatomist of the ancient world, held to the theory of congested 'semen', for be believed that women too produced sperm. Hysteria, he thought, did not affect women who were 'fertile and receptive and eager to the advances of their husbands', but only the sexually continent, whose retained uterine secretions caused bad blood, irritation of the nerves, and finally paroxysms. He confirmed his theory by manipulating the genitals of one of his hysterical patients, a widow: 'There followed twitchings accompanied at the same time by pain and pleasure after which she admitted [*sic*] turbid and abundant sperm. From that time on she was freed of all the evil she felt' (quoted in Veith, 1965, p.38).

Traditional medical theory and practice in the case of hysteria must itself be set in the wider context of professional and popular theorising by men about women. How far was this simply male ideology — ideas designed to justify men's rule — rather than dispassionate inquiry? On the professional side, just as there were disputes between the medical schools of Cos and Cnidus in the fifth century BC, so there was no general agreement between male theorists as to the physical and mental properties of men and women; though they were seen as characteristically different. Here, for example, is a famous statement by the Roman writer Pliny the younger, from the second century AD:

In all genera in which the distinction of male and female is found, Nature makes a similar differentiation in the mental characteristics of the sexes. This differentiation is the most obvious in the case of human kind and in that of the larger animals and the viviparous quadrupeds [four-legged animals that give birth to live young]. In the case of these latter, the female is softer in character, is the sooner tamed, admits more readily of caressing, is more apt in the way of learning .... In all cases, excepting those of the bear and leopard, the female is less spirited than the male, ... softer in disposition, more mischievous, less simple, more impulsive, and more attentive to the nurture of the young; the male, on the other hand, is more spirited than the female, more savage, more simple and less cunning ... the nature of man is most rounded off and complete, and consequently in man the qualities or capacities above referred to are found in their perfection. Hence woman is more compassionate than man, more easily moved to tears, at the same time is more jealous, more querulous, more apt to scold and to strike. She

is, furthermore, more prone to despondency and less hopeful than the man, more void of shame or self-respect, more false of speech, more deceptive, and of more retentive memory. She is also more wakeful, more shrinking, more difficult to rouse to action, and requires a smaller quantity of nutriment. (quoted in Maclean, 1980, p.42)

This analysis of mental qualities was informed by the humoral theory discussed in Chapter 2. The body and the mind were seen in unitary terms and direct physical causes were given for what we would now see as mental states. Women's bodies were seen as cold, damp and burdened with unconsumed waste material — the menstrual flow. They could become volatile, even nasty, if this material were not properly discharged. Humoral theory also accounted for their special virtues. A combination of cold and moist produced a retentive memory, because, like wax, impressions can be registered easily on cold moist substances. Likewise, imagination and inventiveness were thought to be stronger in women because cold and moist substances were held to change their form more readily. The womb itself acted directly on women's mental state. It weakened rationality and increased the incidence and violence of passions in women. Finally, the softer flesh of women predisposed them to psychological softness. Women were, therefore, rather different from men precisely because their bodies were different.

☐ On Pliny's analysis, are women inferior or superior to men?
■ In many respects, Pliny gives each gender virtues that the other lacks. Women are less spirited, but they are also 'more apt in the way of learning', and so on. However, although much of his analysis portrays the character of the two genders as complementary, men are given leadership qualities denied to women. They seem to be bolder, more independent, more cheerful and more straightforward.

Some classical writers stressed women's inferiority more than others. Although Galen believed that women also produced sperm, he did hold that human reproduction was based on seed from both men and women. In this respect, he might be seen as more egalitarian than Aristotle, who believed that children were created from male sperm alone, the woman being merely a receptacle. Aristotle, a Greek philosopher from the fourth century BC, whose father had been a doctor, also conducted biological investigations, and his views on women were cited for generations afterwards. To Aristotle, women were anatomically defective versions of men, 'mutilated males' as he called them. Not only were they biologically inferior, they were, accordingly, morally weaker too.

In the medieval period many male writers took a particularly anti-female, or *misogynist*, stand. One commonly cited work is the anonymous fourteenth-century compendium *De Secretis Mulierum* ('On the Secrets of Women'). This was allegedly written at the request of a priest who sought guidance in assigning a just penance to women for their sins, given that they are 'extremely venemous during their menstrual periods'. It warned, for example, that retained menstrual fluid in old women could have dire effects; a baleful glance from an old woman might, apparently, kill a young child.

This work, however, belongs to a different tradition from those cited earlier. Pliny, Aristotle and Galen all belong to the mainstream of European academic and scientific thought. By contrast, *De Secretis Mulierum* is a compilation of semi-popular lore which draws widely on the European folk tradition as well as on more academic sources. Its particular importance lies in the way it was to become incorporated in the work known for centuries as *Aristotle's Masterpiece*, the most popular work on obstetrics and gynaecology of all time. This work went through hundreds of editions in English between 1684 and 1930, and was probably the most important source of popular information about sexual matters and childbirth. It had, however, little to do with Aristotle and was principally a collection of folklore based on a humoral pathology.

Besides the academic and the folklore traditions, a third important source of theory about the character of men and women was that of religion. Christianity became the official religion of the Roman Empire under Constantine in the early part of the fourth century AD. In the Old Testament, in particular, women have a different place from men. Not only is it Eve who persuades Adam to eat the apple from the Tree of Knowledge, but God punishes them in the following terms:

> Unto the woman he said: 'I will greatly multiply thy sorrow and thy conception; in sorrow thou shalt bring forth children; and thy desire shall be to thy husband, and he shall rule over thee.' And unto Adam he said, 'Because thou hast harkened unto thy wife, and has eaten of the tree, of which I commanded thee, saying, "Thou shalt not eat of it": cursed is the ground for thy sake; in sorrow shalt thou eat of it all the days of thy life; thorns also and thistles shall it bring forth to thee; and thou shalt eat the herb of the field; in the sweat of thy face shalt thou eat bread, till thou return to the ground; for out of it wast thou taken: for dust thou art and unto dust shalt thou return.' (Genesis 3: 16–19, Authorised Version)

Men who wished to do so could therefore ascribe the more painful features of the human condition to the failings of a woman, and could, moreover, cite scriptural authority in their support. In addition, elements of the Christian tradition gave credence to the demonic or supernatural theories of disease which were a standard part of European folklore and this, too, was sometimes used against women. As we saw in Chapter 2, some of the Greek doctors had spoken out strongly in favour of naturalistic theories of illness. The scientific tradition of the classical period, humoral theory, related everything to a physical cause. It claimed, as we saw in Chapter 3, that epilepsy was not a 'sacred disease' but had a purely natural explanation. Likewise, for doctors like Galen, the origin of hysteria had a natural cause — suppressed sexuality.

In the Christian tradition, however, not only were some forms of mental illness thought to be caused by demonic possession, but sexuality itself was viewed by some theologians as supernaturally fraught with evil tendencies and influences. Sexuality is at the heart of The Fall in Genesis. As soon as Adam and Eve have eaten the apple, 'the eyes of them both were opened, and they knew that they were naked; and they sewed fig-leaves together, and made themselves aprons.' (Genesis 3: 7) According to St Augustine, Bishop of Hippo (AD 354–430) and the most influential of the early theologians, 'concupiscence', or sexual lust, was the source of original sin in Adam and Eve.

Such an analysis opens the way to an entirely different account of the origins of hysteria. Whereas doctors like Galen had seen it as the product of sexual continence, some of those in a more Christian tradition came to see it as the product of a demonically inspired lust, whose cure lay in sexual renunciation. In other words, though both sides shared a sexual theory of hysteria, one party sought a cure in sexual fulfilment, the other in sexual abstinence. Both these traditions continued to have a powerful influence throughout the medieval period. However, it is important to remember that, despite the views of the Church Fathers, the medieval period could be far franker than our own about human sexuality and often took a cheerfully matter-of-fact approach to the subject. Here, for example, is Chaucer's description of the Wife of Bath's sexual temperament:

> Venus me yaf my lust, my likerousnesse
> And Mars yaf me my sturdy hardinesse.
> Myn ascendant was Taur and Mars therinne—
> Allas, allas, that evere love was sinne!
> I folwed ay my inclinacioun,
> By vertu of my constellacioun,
> That made me I could nought withdrawe
> My chambre of Venus from a good felawe.
> (Chaucer, *Canterbury Tales*, Wife of Bath's Prologue, late fourteenth century, 611–618; 'yaf' = gave, 'likerousnesse' = lecherousness, 'felawe' = fellow)

□ Yet another traditional analysis of sexuality is offered in this passage. What is it?

■ That of astrology.

There were, then, a variety of conflicting traditions from which those in the medieval world might draw when they theorised about women's nature, about sexuality and, more specifically, about hysteria. Astrology, Graeco-Roman science, European folklore and Christian theology all had a part to play, each influencing the others. Such conflicting traditions continued for many years; indeed, the contemporary analysis of human sexuality and of gender is still riven by many fierce debates. Nevertheless, by the time of the Renaissance, the classical naturalistic theories of Galen began to supersede the supernatural theories of Christian doctrine, at least within the academic tradition. In the sixteenth century, medical practitioners like the Swiss Paracelsus (1493–1541) and the Belgian Johann Weyer (1515–88) argued that hysterical symptoms, epileptic seizures and the like were not the product of demons but were entirely natural products.

Given this return to naturalistic theories, many of the cures recommended for hysteria in the late sixteenth and seventeenth centuries are very similar to those suggested nearly 1 500 years before. William Harvey (1577–1657), whose discovery of the circulation of the blood was one of the outstanding feats of seventeenth-century science, proclaimed that, 'The virtue which proceeds from the male *in coitu* [during intercourse] has such prodigious powers of fecundation that the whole woman, both in mind and body undergoes a change.' (Merchant, 1982, p.161). Most academically trained doctors of this period believed, with Galen, that hysteria, or the '*furor uterinus*' was caused by a woman's retained and corrupted 'seed'. The treatment recommended, for example, by the great surgical pioneer of the sixteenth century, Ambroise Paré (1510–90), followed the standard pattern:

> The sick woman must ... bee placed on her back, haveing her breast and stomach loos; and all her cloaths and garments slack and loos about her, whereby shee may take breath the more easily and shee must be called on by her own name, with a loud voice in her ears; and pulled hard by the hair of the temples and neck, but yet especially by the hairs of the secret parts. (quoted in Bart and Scully, 1979, p.356)

Paré reasoned that by 'provokeing or causing pain in the lower parts' the woman could be 'brought to her self'. At the same time, the foul 'vapour' rising inside her body from the fermenting semen in her womb could be 'drawn downwards' and expelled (Bart and Scully, 1979, p.356).

Ironically, however, this 'victory' of naturalistic theories of hysteria occurred at much the same time as the great European witch-craze of the fifteenth, sixteenth and seventeenth centuries; a wave of persecution and execution which exemplifies some of the more fanatical Church teachings about women, about female sexuality and about supernatural theories. It has already been mentioned in the discussion of Mary Daly's thesis of gynocide and it may possibly overlap with notions of hysteria in a number of ways.

Women and witchcraft

Murdock's survey of the global distribution of theories of disease-causation, cited in Chapter 3, suggests that witchcraft theories are confined to the area around the Mediterranean, Europe, the Near East and the northern half of Africa. The persecution and execution of 'witches', who included a few men but were mostly elderly or unattached women (see Figure 9.2), seems to be an ancient

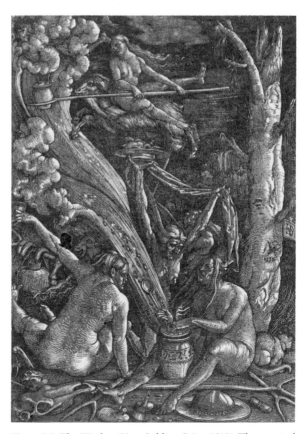

Figure 9.2 The Witches (Hans Balding Grien, 1510). The goat and the cat were associated with women and witchcraft because of their presumed slyness and sexual lust.

tradition in these lands. However, in the late fifteenth and sixteenth centuries there was a major wave of witch-hunting that many, though not all, historians see as shaped by anti-female prejudice.

Intellectual support for this wave of terror was heavily influenced by some of the Church's teachings. A link between the teachings of Aristotle and the religious belief in demonism was made by the highly influential work, the *Canon Episcopi*, in the ninth and tenth centuries. Much later, in 1484, Pope Innocent VIII denounced the treacheries of witchcraft and gave *carte blanche* to the Inquisition, among them the Dominican friars Heinrich Kramer and Jacob Sprenger, who were preparing their treatise *Malleus Maleficarum* ('Hammer of the Witches'). The book appeared in 1486 and, thanks to the new art of printing, proliferated in at least twenty-nine editions. These lay on the benches of magistrates and judges across most of Europe for more than 200 years, though, since it was a Catholic work, it was ignored in Britain and had relatively little influence on Protestant magistrates. Even so, it is generally estimated that around 1 000 executions for witchcraft occurred in England during this period.

Malleus Maleficarum portrays some of the more fanatical medieval teachings about women and female sexuality. Believing with St Augustine that since 'the first corruption of sin ... came to us through the act of generation, ... greater power is allowed by God to the devil in this act than in all others', Kramer and Sprenger concluded

> All witchcraft comes from carnal lust, which is in women insatiable. See *Proverbs xxx*: There are three things that are never satisfied, yea, a fourth thing which says not, It is enough; that is, the mouth of the womb. Wherefore for the sake of fulfilling their lusts they consort even with devils .... It is no matter for wonder that there are more women than men found infected with the heresy of witchcraft. And in consequence of this, it is better called the heresy of witches than of wizards, since the name is taken from the more powerful party. (quoted in Summers, 1971, pp.47–8)

The consorting with devils referred to is described in another passage:

> The witches themselves have often been seen lying on their backs in the fields or the woods, naked up to the very navel, and it has been apparent from the disposition of those limbs and members which pertain to the venereal act and orgasm, as also from the agitation of their legs and thighs, that, all invisibly to the bystanders, they have been copulating with Incubus devils. (quoted in Summers, 1971, p.114)

Finally, here is a description from *Malleus Maleficarum* of 'the formal rules for initiating a process of justice, how it should be conducted, and the method of pronouncing sentence'. After discussing matters relating to judges and witnesses, Kramer and Sprenger turn to the defendant. Her house has been ransacked, her maid-servant or companions locked up, her accusers cross-examined. But she cannot be condemned to death unless convicted by her own confession. So she is to be stripped naked and 'persuaded' by the judge, with 'other honest men zealous for the faith', to 'induce her to confess the truth voluntarily'. 'And if she will not, let him order the officers to bind her with cords, and apply her to some engine of torture.' If she remains silent, the tortures are to be increased, alternating with periods of 'persuasion'. She must not be left alone in the intervals lest the devil cause her to kill herself. Nor may she remain unshaved. The hair must be removed from 'every part' of the witch's body, for 'in order to preserve their power of silence they are in the habit of hiding some superstitious object ... in their hair, or even in the most secret parts of their bodies which must not be named' (quoted in Summers, 1971, pp.222–8).

Hysteria overlaps with the phenomenon of witchcraft in highly complex and controversial ways (Spanos and Gottlieb, 1979). Church doctrines about the evils of sexuality, particularly female sexuality, are one obvious example. It might also be that some of the women tried as witches were themselves hysterical: the descriptions of some of the characteristic signs of witches parallel some later descriptions of the symptoms of hysteria; symptoms such as local immunities from pain, curious skin disorders, hallucinations, false pregnancies, suicide attempts and frigidity. On the other hand, hysteria might itself be seen as the product of others' witchcraft. Finally, it is at least possible to describe the activities of those engaged in the persecution of 'witches' as itself an example of mass hysteria.

Masculine anatomy

The resurgence during the Renaissance of the European belief in witches should remind us that what we may now see as progress is rarely a straightforward matter. Scientific advance in one part of the society is matched by barbarism in another. Moreover, the naturalistic explanations produced by the new science could be just as misogynist in character as the demonic theories, though with somewhat less appalling consequences. Nonetheless, the appeal to natural rather than supernatural explanations was a major advance and was matched, in its turn, by a systematic exploration of the human body, something that was eventually to have profound consequences for theories of hysteria. Since humoral theory held that mental states were the direct product of physical states, the detailed explanation of human physiology and anatomy held out

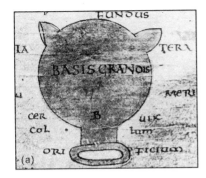

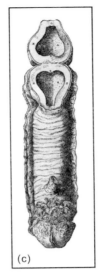

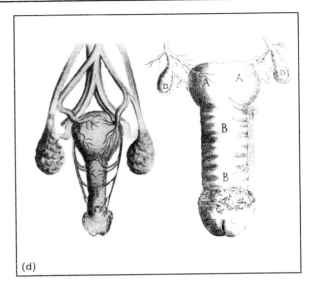

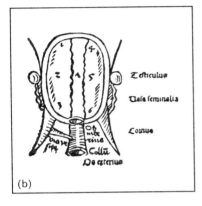

Figure 9.3 (a) The uterus in a ninth-century manuscript, with the 'fundus' or base, the cervix, the neck or vagina (*collam*) and the vaginal mouth (*avificiam*), all roughly labelled. (b) A sixteenth century illustration of the uterus copied from the *Anathomia* (1316) of Mondino dei Luzzi. (c) The uterus, vagina and external genitalia. (Andreas Vesalius, 1543) (d) The female reproductive organs according to Georg Bartisch, 1575, (left) and Scipione Mercurio, 1595, (right).

the promise of a better scientific understanding of puzzling conditions like hysteria. Let us now, therefore, consider the new findings about the traditional seat of hysteria — the womb. Renaissance scientists explored the womb, as they did other parts of the body, with all the tenacity of their contemporaries who turned their instruments of discovery upon the heavens. And, like the astronomers, they made some startling discoveries; for traditional anatomy had been grossly inaccurate.

☐ Consider the anatomical illustrations in Figure 9.3a–d. These appeared originally in documents written by male physicians between the ninth and the sixteenth centuries. Compare them with the modern illustration in Figure 9.4. What differences can you spot between the old and the new versions? What might have been the model for the traditional anatomy?

■ Several errors are perpetuated in the illustrations; for example, the womb includes the cervix and vagina (Figure 9.3a and b) and itself consists of up to seven cavities (Figure 9.3b–d). The ovaries are labelled 'testiculus' (Figure 9.3b), after the male sexual glands, and the urethra is shown opening into the vagina (Figures 9.3a–d). Finally, there can be no mistaking the masculine appearance given to the female reproductive organs in Figure 9.3c and d. This would suggest that male physicians believed women to be formed on the

pattern of men's anatomy, either because of male prejudice, or because, in the absence of detailed anatomical investigation, the only visible model was that of the male reproductive organs.

Until Mondino dei Luzzi (*c*.1275–1326), with the assistance of Alessandra Giliani, dissected two female corpses in 1315–16, anatomists were largely ignorant of the structure

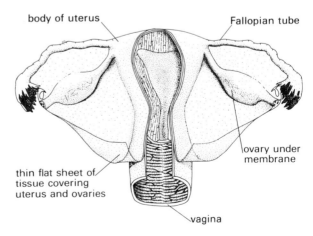

Figure 9.4 A modern anatomical drawing of the female reproductive organs.

of the female generative organs. The fifteenth century saw the first description of the hymen; in the sixteenth century it was realised that the womb was divided into an upper and lower part and that the upper portion is a single cavity. It also saw the first descriptions of the mons veneris and the clitoris, and the first encyclopaedia, or 'system', of gynaecology. In the seventeenth century, the term 'gynaecology' was first used in its several variations; the 'female testicles' were first called ovaries; and the age-old method of describing the female genitalia from the inside out, by beginning with the womb, was reversed. Now anatomical writers began with the external genitalia and worked from the outside in. One recent scholar, Ian Maclean, concluded after a fairly exhaustive study of the literature: 'By 1600, in nearly all medical circles . . . one sex is no longer thought to be an imperfect and incomplete version of the other. Indeed, far from being described as an inferior organ, the uterus now evokes admiration and eulogy for its remarkable role in procreation' (Maclean, 1980, p.33).

Despite this, many of the old anatomical beliefs still lingered on. When, in 1636, John Sadler, 'doctor in physicke' at Norwich, produced a gynaecological handbook for women, *The Sicke Woman's Private Looking Glass*, he wrote that 'the forme or figure of it [the womb] is like a virall member, onley this excepted, the manhood is outward, and the womanhood within' (Sadler, 1636, p.5). Moreover, the womb was still seen as the centre of women's physical and emotional life. Along with the vast majority of seventeenth-century physicians, Sadler held that women's health was determined primarily by the state of their wombs.

> For through the evill quality thereof, the heart, the liver, and the braine are affected; from whence the actions vitall, natural, & animal are hurt; and the virtues concoctive, sanguifficative, distributive, attractive, expulsive, retentive, with all the rest are all weakened. So that from the wombe comes convulsions, epilepsies, apoplexies, palseyes, hecticke fevers, dropsies, malignant ulcers, and to bee short, there is no disease so ill but may procede from the evill quality of it. (Sadler, 1636, preface)

Likewise, although both Soranus and Galen had denied that the womb could move about the body as far back as the second century AD, there were still some seventeenth century physicians who believed this. Jean Liebault, for example, wrote of how the womb:

> often changes position, and makes curious and so to speak, petulant movements in the woman's body. These movements are various: to wit, ascending, descending, convulsive, vagrant, prolapsed. The

womb rises to the liver, spleen, diaphragm, stomach, breast, heart, lung, gullet and head. (quoted in Foucault, 1973, p.144)

Nevertheless, the new anatomy was radically to change the traditional theories of hysteria. Once it was known precisely how the womb was anchored inside the body, it was far harder to imagine it wandering about at will. Moreover, as knowledge of the entire body progressed, the uterus itself, whether moving or stable, was progressively displaced both as the seat of hysteria and as the major cause of female disease. Other parts of the body now came to be seen as playing a major role. The English doctor Thomas Willis (1621–75) is usually credited with the first major critique of uterine theories:

> If a disease of unknown nature and hidden origin appears in a woman in such a manner that its cause escapes us, and that the therapeutic course is uncertain, we immediately blame the bad influence of the uterus, which, for the most part, is not responsible . . . . (quoted in Foucault, 1973, p.138)

Willis still saw the uterus as playing a major role in the production of hysteria, but he thought the condition itself was far less common than tradition made out, and he also believed that the brain too played a major part; indeed, he listed hysteria under diseases of the head. On his analysis, the uterus no longer moved; instead, it made its influence felt on the brain via the humoral fluids and the nervous system. The first beginnings of a shift to a mental as well as a physical explanation occur here.

This basic pattern of new anatomical and physiological discoveries gradually modifying the explanation of hysteria was to be repeated throughout the eighteenth and most of the nineteenth centuries. Herman Boerhaave (1668–1738), the Dutch physician and chemist, favoured a humoral explanation of hysteria and pictured it as a condition in which the bodily fluids became so volatile that they were agitated by the least movement. However, with the general decline in humoral theories following the detailed exploration of muscle by the Swiss physiologist Albrecht von Haller (1708–77), there was a new vogue for theories of disease which focused on bodily solids rather than fluids. The analysis of hysteria likewise changed. It was now argued that strong men never became hysterical and labouring women only rarely because their bodies were strong and dense. By contrast, so it was claimed, hysteria was rife amongst delicate upper-class women who led a soft, idle, luxurious life.

    □   What evidence is there to support this observation that working-class women were less vulnerable to hysteria?

■ None. Neither Briquet's nineteenth-century data nor those of Smith-Rosenberg suggest any significant variation in class incidence.

The shift towards mental explanations became increasingly prominent in the eighteenth century. The gradual exploration of the nervous system led to the belief that it was here that the answer to the mystery of hysteria lay. A woman with 'too much feeling, . . . an excessive solidarity' with her environment and the beings around her, necessarily fell physically — hysterically — ill. Her passions and imaginations had been cultivated too complacently; nervous impressions had overcharged her mind. The problem lay in part with an over-sensitive nervous system. Such women were said to be 'nervous', 'irritable', or suffering from excessive 'sensibility'. Such a state is one of the topics of Jane Austen's novel *Sense and Sensibility* (1811). Marianne, one of the central characters, is portrayed as physically and mentally vulnerable. An infection almost carries her off at one point in the novel, and throughout much of the story she swings from one mood to another: excessively happy, or excessively glum. Here, for example, is how she reacts to the news that someone to whom her sister, Elinor, is attached has married another, 'Marianne gave a violent start, fixed her eyes upon Elinor, saw her turning pale, and fell back in her chair in hysterics.' (Austen, 1969, p.343). And here is another report of her from an earlier scene in the novel:

> 'Poor Marianne!' said her brother to Colonel Brandon in a low voice, as soon as he could secure his attention, — 'She has not such good health as her sister, — she is very nervous, — she has not Elinor's constitution; — and one must allow that there is something very trying to a young woman who *has been* a beauty, in the loss of her personal attractions. You would not think it perhaps, but Marianne *was* remarkably handsome a few months ago; quite as handsome as Elinor. — Now you see it is all gone.' (Austen, 1969, p.242, emphases as in original)

□ Austen portrays Marianne's brother as making allowances for her hysterics. However, she also hints at another explanation besides those offered by her brother. What is it?

■ She implies that the cause lies partly in the way the world and particularly men, evaluate women.

Fully developed social theories of hysteria were not, however, produced until the twentieth century. Before this time, medical inquiry was still focused primarily upon the body, though as we have seen the site of its investigation underwent major changes. By the nineteenth century, the search was focused primarily on the brain. In the long trail of inquiry, medicine had moved from the womb, via the fluids and solids and the nervous system to the most complex of all the body's organs. As we saw in Chapter 8, even this inquiry was to prove fruitless. In the latter half of the nineteenth century, and even more so in this century, doctors and social scientists turned instead to other areas of investigation. Mental and social theories came to dominate the field; the unconscious with Freud; social circumstances (and heredity) with Briquet; gender relationships with Smith-Rosenberg. And some came to deny the existence or validity of the phenomenon altogether.

The various changes should not, however, blind us to the way in which traditional beliefs have lingered on. The Egyptian belief in the wandering womb, though apparently put to rest by the new anatomy, still found an echo in Victorian 'uterine displacement' theory, and Galen's belief in the importance of congestion was also paralleled in this era in the notion that uterine 'inflammation' was a primal cause of female maladies, including hysteria. Many of the old treatments remained. A 'moderate number' of leeches to the neck of the uterus was supposed to cure convulsions by restoring the organ to 'a state of integrity', although sometimes, doctors maintained, 'nothing but the application of the most powerful caustics, the acid nitrate of mercury, or the potassa cum calce, so modifies the vitality of the part as radically to cure the inflammation' (Bennet, 1853, pp.261, 269, 417).

Finally, note that, although the explanatory base of hysteria has continually shifted as medical knowledge and theory changed, women themselves have kept on being blamed. Just as Aristotle believed that women were biologically inferior, so the eighteenth-century theory that located the problem directly in the nerves, in excessive female sensitivity, also held that certain social pursuits might bring on the condition. Novel-reading, theatre-going, intellectual ambition, and above all an immoderate interest in sex — such 'unnatural' abuses had brought about their natural effect, and the individual was morally accountable. Even the more modern mental or social theories of hysteria contain some potential for blaming the hysterical woman. If the condition is viewed from the perspective of the sick role, it may still be argued that the woman is exploiting the role unfairly. Likewise, though supernatural theories have disappeared from professional medical analysis, they still find an echo in some of the ways in which women are viewed in our culture. Cecil Helman argued that popular discussion of 'germs' carried with it a flavour of the traditional belief in invisible malignant spirits. In similar fashion, the demonic view of female sexuality still lingers. The medieval dichotomy between the Virgin Mary on the one hand and the insatiable woman on the other is repeated both in the Victorian division between the 'angel in the house' and the 'fallen woman' and in the double-standard of sexual morality which still applies today.

Objectives for Chapter 9

When you have studied this chapter, you should be able to:

9.1 Describe the way that male theories of women have served to control women as well as to understand them.

9.2 Describe the development of physical explanations of hysteria and their eventual replacement with mental explanations.

9.3 Describe the long survival of ancient professional and popular male views of women.

Questions for Chapter 9

1 (*Objective 9.1*) In what ways could God's speech to Eve and Adam (cited in this chapter) be seen as a masculine ideology; something to be used by men in their relationships with women?

2 (*Objective 9.2*) 'Beyond what we may call the exterior man, who is composed of parts which are visible to the senses, there is an interior man formed of a system of animal spirits, a man who can be seen only with the eyes of the mind. This latter man, closely joined and so to speak united with the corporeal constitution, is more or less deranged from his state to the degree that the principles which form the machine have a natural firmness. That is why this disease [hysteria] attacks women more than men because they have a more delicate, less firm constitution, because they lead a softer life and because they are accustomed to the luxuries and commodities of life and not to suffering.' (a late seventeenth-century/early eighteenth-century description quoted in Foucault, 1973, p.149)

(a) In what respects might this be a biological or a mental theory of hysteria?

(b) Does the analysis suggest that women are to blame?

3 (*Objective 9.3*) 'The frequency of intercourse depends entirely on the male sex drive .... The bride should be advised to allow her husband's sex drive to set their pace and she should attempt to gear hers satisfactorily to his. If she finds after several months or years that this is not possible, she is advised to consult her physician as soon as she realizes there is a real problem. In assuming this role of follow the leader, however, she is cautioned not to make her sexual relations entirely passive .... She may be reminded that it is unsatisfactory to take a tone-deaf individual to a concert.' (*Novak's Textbook of Gynecology*, quoted in Scully, 1980, p.111)

(a) When do you think this was written?

(b) Compare this gynaecological treatment of male and female sexuality with the theories of Galen and Harvey discussed earlier in this chapter.

10
Conclusion

Three final points on which to close: first, some more thoughts on the nature of science; second, a note on an important method of analysis; third, a comment on the biosocial nature of health and disease.

This book began with the vision of Renaissance science. In that dream, humankind was to be 'so firm of mind and purpose as resolutely to sweep away all theories and common notions, and to apply the understanding, thus made fair and even, to a fresh examination of particulars'. By this means, Bacon hoped 'to restore and exalt the power and dominion of man himself, of the human race over the universe' (quoted in Johnston, 1974, p.vii). In other words, science might be able to conquer all, including disease.

The method that Bacon praised, 'the fresh examination of particulars' — that is, reductionism, or getting out and examining the fine detail of the world — has, as he foresaw, proved enormously powerful; the progressive localisation of pathology has enabled many dramatic advances in the scientific understanding and treatment of disease. And as science has progressed, so its own status has risen to a point where Bacon's own estimation of its worth, cited below, is now a common one.

> In the Scriptures, King Solomon, though blessed with empire, gold, splendour of architecture, satellites, servants, ministers and slaves of every kind and degree, with a fleet to boot and a glorious name, and with the flattering admiration of the world, yet prided himself on none of these things. Instead, he declared that, 'It was the glory of God to conceal a thing, the glory of a King to find it out' ... And indeed, it is this glory of discovery that is the true ornament of mankind. In contrast with civil business it never harmed any man, never burdened a conscience with remorse. Its blessing and reward is without ruin, wrong or wretchedness to any. For light is in itself pure and innocent; it may be wrongly used, but cannot in its nature defile. (quoted in Johnston, 1974, p.ix)

Yet, as we have seen, this is not the whole story. Medical science is a magnificent human accomplishment; it is not, however, quite as innocent as Bacon suggests.

☐ What criticisms might you now make of Bacon's assumptions in the quotations cited above?

■ You might have questioned (i) how far Bacon intended the 'power and dominion of man' to refer to men rather than women; (ii) whether it was either possible or appropriate to exalt such dominion over the 'universe'; (iii) whether the 'blessing and reward' of science is really 'without ruin, wrong or wretchedness to any'. The advantages of hysterectomy, a blessing of science, are much disputed by some and one may ask how far 'empire and gold' are in fact bound closely to science and its application. Bacon admits that science can be wrongly used, but this is a mere footnote to his paean of praise.

You have seen other things too. Not only may science be 'wrongly used', but its powers to do good may also, on occasion, be exaggerated. As you have seen, there is some reason to question precisely how far biomedical science has contributed to the enormous progress in human health that has been made over the last century or two.* Science, as applied to navigation, engineering and agriculture, may perhaps have made more of a contribution to human health than has biomedical science.

Remember, too, one other criticism of the Whig version of medical history. Montaigne's scepticism about the very possibility of doctors possessing useful knowledge has certainly been shown to be wrong. Nevertheless, he was right about one central point. Health and disease are matters of enormous complexity. It was not until the nineteenth century, after more than 300 years of scientific investigation, that European medical science really took off. Moreover, although it now has many important achievements to its credit, there is still much that is obscure. The causes of the great pandemics of bubonic plague, the nature of hysteria, the determinants of hysterectomy — all these are the subject of enormous debate. And such debates are to be found in every aspect of health, disease and medicine. Even in an apparently straightforward triumph,

---

* This analysis is taken much further in *The Health of Nations*.

such as that over pernicious anaemia, vital aspects of the condition remain unknown. Medical science may have progressed since Montaigne and Bacon, but it still has far to go.

How then should this complexity be tackled, if further progress is to be made? This brings us to our second topic. The methods that Bacon suggested, the caution and the focus on detail — the 'fresh examination of particulars' — both these continue to have great power. There is, however, one further method which has not so far been mentioned, though it has been drawn on extensively in the preparation of this book. Much of what you have read in this book has been taken from history and anthropology. Some of you may have wondered why it is necessary to spend so much time studying people who live or lived in times and places remote from our own. Why study people whose way of life is so different, whose knowledge is so apparently bizarre? The answer is that we cannot properly understand our own medical knowledge, our own approach to health and disease, unless we place it in a *comparative* social context. It is only through comparison with other human beings in other times and places that we can understand the ways in which we ourselves are unique, and the ways in which we are the same. Implicitly, of course, we make such comparisons all the time. Phrases like 'the modern British health service' or 'health and disease in modern Britain' carry with them a number of crucial but normally hidden suggestions. The word 'modern' suggests that there is something distinctive about the way we now think and act; something radically different from, even superior, to previous eras. And 'British' implies that that society is rather different from any other; that it has its own special characteristics. If you are British, it too often conveys an assumption of national superiority. All these assumptions need checking carefully. Most of us live in an extraordinarily parochial world, a world which rarely inspects its past or its neighbours in any serious way. But it is only through such comparison that we can hope to understand the complexities of health, disease and medical knowledge; can judge the many changes that have been made and appreciate the more universal aspects of the human condition.

The third and final point concerns one particular comparison — that of plague, hysterectomy and hysteria. Plague stands at the biological end of the biosocial spectrum. It is immediately and self-evidently a disease — there can be no mistaking plague if you happen to catch it. It affects a very high proportion of those in its path, pretty much regardless of their rank or condition, and a central part of the origin of plague epidemics would seem to lie in biological mutation.

☐ Hysteria and hysterectomy seem to stand more towards the social end of the biosocial spectrum. How do they differ in this respect from plague?

■ First, plague is clearly a disease, but there is considerable disagreement over whether either hysteria or some of the conditions used as indications for hysterectomy should be considered as diseases. Plague is easy to diagnose, but different doctors use very different criteria in diagnosing hysteria and select different indications in recommending hysterectomy. Such decisions seem to be far more strongly shaped by social and economic forces than is true of plague. Second, hysteria may possibly have a largely social cause — something that is certainly not true of plague.

There are, therefore, major differences in the manner in which different diseases are shaped by biological and social factors. The overall influence of each also varies. Despite this, some of the partisans of the biological sciences seek to explain everything in biological terms. Such attempts are as futile as those made by their counterparts in the social sciences. Sometimes one explanation fits a problem better, sometimes the other, and there is always something that each side can contribute. In the long run, only a joint approach can hope to succeed.

References and further reading

References

ARMITAGE, KAREN, J., SCHNEIDERMAN, LAWRENCE, J. and BASS, ROBERT, A. (1979) Response of physicians to medical complaints in men and women, *Journal of the American Medical Association*, **241**, pp.2 186–7.

ASHTON, JOHN and EDWARDS, GUY (1980) Marching bands and mass hysteria, *New Society*, 24 July, pp.166–7.

AUSTEN, JANE (1969) *Sense and Sensibility*, Penguin (first published in 1811).

BART, PAULINE and SCULLY, DIANA (1979) The politics of hysteria: the case of the wandering womb, in E.F. Gomberg and V. Franks (eds) *Gender and Disordered Behaviour: Sex Differences in Psychopathology*, Bruner/ Mazel, New York, pp.354–80.

BENNET, J.H. (1853) *A Practical Treatise on Inflammation of the Uterus, its Cervix and Appendages and its Connexion with Uterine Disease*, 3rd edn, John Churchill, London (first edition in 1845).

BIRABEN, JEAN-NOEL (1975) *Les Hommes et la Peste* (2 vols) Mouton, The Hague.

BLACK, NICK, BOSWELL, DAVID, GRAY, ALASTAIR, MURPHY, SEAN and POPAY, JENNIE (eds) (1984) *Health and Disease: A Reader*, The Open University Press. The Course Reader.

BOCCACCIO (1855) *The Decameron*, trans. W.K. Kelly, Bohn, London.

BRADLEY, LESLIE (1977) The most famous of all English plagues: a detailed analysis of the plague at Eyam 1665–6, in *The Plague Reconsidered*, Local Population Studies, Fourth Supplement, pp.63–94.

British Medical Journal (1976) The search for a psychiatric Esperanto (Editorial) 11 September, pp.600–1.

British Medical Journal (1977) Hysterectomy and sterilisation: changes of fashion and mind (Editorial), 17 September, pp.715–6.

CARPENTER, EDWARD (1916) *My Days and Dreams: Being Autobiographical Notes*, George Allen and Unwin.

CASS, V. (1982) Letter to *Good Housekeeping* ('You Write To Us') June, pp.40–1.

CHODOFF, PAUL (1974) The diagnosis of hysteria: an overview, *American Journal of Psychiatry*, **131**, pp.1 073–8.

CHODOFF, PAUL (1982) Hysteria and women, *American Journal of Psychiatry*, **139**, pp.545–51.

CHRISTIE, A.B. (1983) Plague, in *Oxford Textbook of Medicine*, D.J. Weatherall, J.G.G. Ledingham and D.A. Warrell (eds), Oxford University Press, pp.5.205–10.

COHEN, MANDEL, E., ROBINS, ELI, PURTELL, JAMES, J., ALTMANN, MARTHA, W. and REID, DUNCAN, E. (1953) Excessive surgery in hysteria, *Journal of the American Medical Association*, **151**, pp.977–86.

COLLIGAN, MICHAEL, J. and MURPHY, LAWRENCE, R. (1982) A review of mass psychogenic illness in work settings, in M.J. Colligan, J.W. Pennebaker and L.R. Murphy (eds) *Mass Psychogenic Illness*, Lawrence Erlbaum Associates, Hillsdale, New Jersey, pp.33–52.

CRAWFURD, R. (1914) *Plague and Pestilence in Literature and Art*, Oxford University Press.

CREIGHTON, CHARLES (1894) *History of Epidemics in Britain*, Cambridge University Press (Repr. Cass, 1965).

DALY, MARY (1979) *Gyn/Ecology: The Metaethics of Radical Feminism*, The Women's Press.

DEFOE, DANIEL (1902) *A Journal of the Plague Year*, Everyman edition. First published in 1722.

DEWHURST, KENNETH (1966) *Dr. Thomas Sydenham (1624–1689): His Life and Original Writings*, The Wellcome Historical Library, London.

EVANS-PRITCHARD, E.E. (1934) Zande therapeutics, in E.E. Evans-Pritchard *et al. Essays Presented to C.G. Seligman*, Kegan, Paul, Trench, Trubner and Co., pp.49–61.

FOUCAULT, MICHEL (1973) *Madness and Civilisation*, Vintage Books.

FRIEDELL, E. (1927) *Kulturgesicht der Neuzit* (2 vols), Munich.

FULDER, STEPHEN and MONRO, ROBIN (1981) *The Status of Complementary Medicine in the United Kingdom*, Threshold Foundation.

GATH, DENNIS, COOPER, PETER and DAY, ANN (1982) Hysterectomy and psychiatric disorder: I. Levels of psychiatric morbidity before and after hysterectomy, *British Journal of Psychiatry*, **140**, pp.335–50.

GATH, D., OSBORN, M., COOPER, P. and BUNGAY, G. (1984) 'Gynaecological and psychiatric health amongst women in the community', in preparation.

GOTTFRIED, R.S. (1978) *Epidemic Disease in Fifteenth Century England*, Leicester University Press.

HALEY, BRUCE (1978) *The Healthy Body and Victorian Culture*, Harvard University Press.

HATCHER, JOHN (1977) *Plague, Population and the English Economy 1348–1530*, Macmillan.

HELLERSTEIN, E.O., HUME, L.P. and OFFEN, K.M. (eds) (1981) *Victorian Women: A Documentary Account of Women's Lives in Nineteenth Century England, France and the United States*, Harvester, Brighton.

HERZLICH, CLAUDINE (1973) *Health and Illness*, trans. H.D. Graham, Academic Press.

HIRST, L.F. (1953) *The Conquest of Plague*, Oxford University Press.

JAMES, T.B. (1983) *Southampton Sources 1086–1900*, Southampton Records Series XXVI.

JEWSON, N.D. (1976) The disappearance of the sick man from the medical cosmology 1770–1870, *Sociology*, **10**(2), pp.225–44.

JOHNSTON, ARTHUR (1974) Introduction to *Francis Bacon's 'The Advancement of Learning' and 'New Atlantis'*, Oxford University Press.

KESSEL, NEIL and COPPEN, ALEC (1963) The prevalence of common menstrual symptoms, *The Lancet*, 13 July, pp.61–4.

KROLL, PHILIP, CHAMBERLAIN, KENNETH, R. and HALPERN, JAMES (1979) The diagnosis of Briquet's Syndrome in a male population: the veteran's administration revisited, *Journal of Nervous and Mental Disease*, **167**, pp.171–4.

LAUGHLIN, WILLIAM, S. (1977) Acquisition of anatomical knowledge by ancient man, in D. Landy (ed.) *Culture, Disease and Healing*, Macmillan, pp.254–64.

LEBRA, TAKIE SUGIYAMA (1977) Religious conversion and elimination of the sick role, in D. Landy (ed.) *Culture, Disease and Healing*, Macmillan, pp.408–14.

LEESON, JOYCE and GRAY, JUDITH (1978) *Women and Medicine*, Tavistock, London.

LERNER, HARRIET (1974) The hysterical personality: a woman's disease, *Comprehensive Psychiatry*, **15**, pp.157–64.

LLOYD, G.E.R. (ed.) (1978) *Hippocratic Writings*, Penguin.

MACLEAN, IAN (1980) *The Renaissance Notion of Woman*, Cambridge University Press.

MCNEILL, WILLIAM, H. (1979) *Plagues and People*, Penguin.

MCPHERSON, K., STRONG, P., EPSTEIN, A. and JONES, L. (1981) Regional variations in the use of common surgical procedures: within and between England and Wales, Canada and the United States, *Social Science and Medicine*, **15A**, pp.273–88.

MAI, FRANCOIS, M. (1980) Briquet's treatise on hysteria: a synopsis and commentary, *Archives of General Psychiatry*, **37**, pp.1401–5.

MERCHANT, CAROLINE (1982) *The Death of Nature: Women, Ecology and The Scientific Revolution*, Wildwood House.

MILLER, NORMAN, F. (1946) Hysterectomy: therapeutic necessity or surgical racket? *American Journal of Obstetrics and Gynecology*, **51**, pp.804–10.

MINER, HORACE (1956) Body ritual among the Nacirema, *American Anthropologist*, **58**, pp.503–7.

MONTAIGNE, MICHEL DE (1580) Of the resemblances of children to their fathers, *Essays* Book II, Chapter 37. First published 1580; trans. D.M. Frame (1948), Stanford University Press.

MONTAIGNE, MICHEL DE (1952) Upon some verses of Virgil, *Essays* Book III, Chapter 5, Encyclopaedia Britannica, trans. Charles Cotton.

MORRIS, CHRISTOPHER (1977) Plague in Britain, in *The Plague Reconsidered*, Local Population Studies, Fourth Supplement, pp.37–47.

MURDOCK, G.P. (1980) *Theories of Illness: A World Survey*, University of Pittsburgh Press.

NORRIS, JOHN (1977) East or West? The geographic origin of the Black Death, *Bulletin of the History of Medicine*, **51**, p.8.

PARSONS, TALCOTT (1951) *The Social System*, Routledge & Kegan Paul.

PETTY, WILLIAM   (1667) cited in *The Plague Reconsidered*, Local Population Studies, Fourth Supplement, 1977, p.18.

PHILLIPS, ANGELA and RAKUSEN, JILL   (1978) *Our Bodies Ourselves: A Health Book By and For Women* (British edition of the book by the Boston Women's Health Collective), Penguin.

PROCOPIUS   (1914) *Procopius Books 1 and 2*, trans. H.B. Dewing, Loeb Classical Library.

QUINTON, ANTHONY   (1980) *Francis Bacon*, Oxford University Press.

RAWLINGS, AUDREY   (1982) Letter to *Good Housekeeping* ('You Write To Us'), June, p.39.

RIVAZ, G.E.   (1982) Letter to *Good Housekeeping* ('You Write To Us'), June, p.40.

RUSSELL, J.C.   (1948) *British Medieval Population*, University of New Mexico.

SADLER, JOHN   (1636) *The Sick Woman's Private Looking Glass*, printed by Anne Griffin, London.

SCHOFIELD, ROGER   (1977) An anatomy of an epidemic: Colyton, November 1645 to November 1646, in *The Plague Reconsidered*, Local Population Studies, Fourth Supplement, pp.95–126.

SCHULMAN, SAM and SMITH, ANNE   (1963) The concept of health among Spanish-speaking villagers of New Mexico and Colorado, *Journal of Health and Social Behaviour*, 4, pp.226–34.

SCULLY, DIANA   (1980) *Men Who Control Women's Health: The Miseducation of Obstetrician-Gynecologists*, Houghton Mifflin, Boston.

SELWOOD, TOM and WOOD, CARL   (1978) Incidence of hysterectomy in Australia, *Medical Journal of Australia*, 2, pp.201–4.

SHREWSBURY, J.F.D.   (1971) *A History of Bubonic Plague in the British Isles*, Cambridge University Press.

SHRYOCK, RICHARD   (1979) *The Development of Modern Medicine*, University of Wisconsin Press. First edition 1936.

SIGERIST, HENRY   (1977) The special position of the sick, in D. Landy (ed.) *Culture, Disease and Healing: Studies in Medical Anthropology*, Macmillan.

SKEY, F.C.   (1867) *Hysteria*, Longmans, Green, Reader and Dyer.

SLACK, PAUL   (1977) The local incidence of epidemic disease: the case of Bristol 1540–1650, in *The Plague Reconsidered*, Local Population Studies, Fourth Supplement, pp.49–62.

SLACK, PAUL   (1981) The disappearance of plague: an alternative view, *Economic History Review*, 34, p.476.

SLATER, ELIOT   (1965) Diagnosis of 'hysteria', *British Medical Journal*, 29 May, pp.1 395–9.

SMITH, REA   (1922) The unnecessary operation, *Surgery, Gynecology and Obstetrics*, 35, pp.820–3.

SMOLLET, TOBIAS   (1967) *Humphrey Clinker*, Penguin. First published 1771.

SPANOS, NICHOLAS P. and GOTTLIEB, JACK   (1979) Demonic possession, mesmerism and hysteria: a social psychological perspective on their historical interpretation, *Journal of Abnormal Psychology*, 88(5), pp.527–46.

STARR, PAUL   (1982) *The Social Transformation of American Medicine*, Basic Books, New York.

SULLOWAY, FRANK, J.   (1980) *Freud: Biologist of the Mind*, Fontana.

SUMMERS, M. (trans. and ed.)   (1971) *The Malleus Maleficarum of Heinrich Kramer and James Sprenger*, Dover Publications, New York.

THE CHEMIST AND DRUGGIST   (1898) *Diseases and Remedies*, London.

The Lancet   (1977) What every woman needs to know (Editorial), 29 January, p.232.

TURNER, E.S.   (1958) *Call The Doctor: A Social History Of Medical Men*, Michael Joseph.

VAYDA, EUGENE, MINDELL, WILLIAM, R. and RUTKOW, IRA, M.   (1982) A decade of surgery in Canada, England, Wales and the United States, *Archives of Surgery*, 117, p.846.

VEITH, I.   (1965) *Hysteria: The History of a Disease*, University of Chicago Press.

VESSEY, MARTIN, P., CLARKE, J.A. and MACKENZIE, I.Z.   (1979) Dilatation and curettage in young women, *Health Bulletin*, March, pp.59–62.

WILDE, OSCAR   (1954) *The Importance of Being Earnest*, Penguin.

WILLIAMS, RORY   (1983) Concepts of health: an analysis of lay logic, *Sociology*, 17, pp.185–205.

WILMOTH, J.   (1982) Letter to *Good Housekeeping* ('You Write To Us'), June, p.39.

WOODRUFF, ROBERT, A., CLAYTON, P.J. and GUZE, S.B.   (1971) Hysteria: studies of diagnosis, outcome and prevalence, *Journal of the American Medical Association*, 18 January, pp.425–8.

WRIGHT, RALPH, C.   (1969) Hysterectomy: past, present and future, *Obstetrics and Gynecology*, 33(4), pp.560–3.

ZIEGLER, PHILIP   (1970) *The Black Death*, Pelican.

ZELDIN, THEODORE   (1973) *France 1848–1945*, vol. 1, Oxford University Press.

Further reading

An excellent collection of historical and contemporary articles which covers many of the topics in this book is:

CAPLAN, ARTHUR, L., ENGLEHARDT, JR, TRISTRAM, H. and McCARTNEY, JAMES, J. (eds) (1981) *Concepts of Health and Disease: Interdisciplinary Perspectives*, Addison-Wesley.

Chapter 2

SHRYOCK, RICHARD (1979) *The Development of Modern Medicine*, University of Wisconsin Press. First edition 1936.
Although written more than forty years ago, this remains the classic text on the development of medical science.

Chapter 3

LANDY, DAVID (1983) Medical anthropology: a critical appraisal, in Julio L. Ruffini (ed.) *Advances in Medical Social Science*, Gordon and Breach, pp.185–314.
This detailed overview is the best guide to medical anthropology.

Chapters 4–6

HATCHER, JOHN (1977) *Plague, Population and Economy 1348–1530*, Macmillan.
A detailed study of the impact of plague on the English economy.

McNEILL, WILLIAM, H. (1979) *Plagues and People*, Penguin.
A well-written survey of the impact of infectious disease on human history.

Chapters 8 and 9

GELDER, MICHAEL, GATH, DENNIS and MAYOU, RICHARD (1983) *The Oxford Textbook of Psychiatry*, Oxford University Press.
This book includes a clear review of both hysteria and hypochondria from the standpoint of mainstream British psychiatry.

JORDANOVA, LUDI (1981) Natural facts: a historical perspective on science and sexuality, in C.P. MacCormack and M. Strathern (eds) *Nature, Culture and Gender*, Cambridge University Press, pp.42–69.
This article is a good general review from a feminist position.

Acknowledgements

Grateful acknowledgement is made to the following sources for material used in this book:

Text
T. Zeldin, *France 1848–1945*, vol. 1, Oxford University Press, 1973; H. Miner, Body ritual among the Nacirema, in *American Anthropologist*, vol. 58, no. 3, The American Anthropological Association, 1956.

Tables
Table 3.1 S. Fulder and R. Munro, *The Status of Complementary Medicine in the UK*, Research Council for Complementary Medicine, 1981; *Table 7.1* N. Kessen and A. Coppen, The prevalence of common menstrual symptoms, in *The Lancet*, July 13, 1963; *Table 7.2* D. Gath *et al.*, Gynaecological and psychiatric health amongst women in the community, unpub.; *Table 7.3* D. Gath *et al.*, Hysterectomy and psychiatric disorder: I, in *British Journal of Psychiatry*, vol. 140, 1982; *Table 8.2* P. Kroll *et al.*, Diagnosis of Briquet's Syndrome in a male population, in *Journal of Nervous and Mental Disease*, vol. 167, Williams and Wilkins Co., 1979.

Figures
Frontispiece, by permission of the Librarian, Glasgow University Library; *Figures 2.1 and 6.4* Mary Evans Picture Library; *Figures 2.2, 4.1 and 7.2* Punch; *Figures 2.3, 2.4, 2.7 and 5.4* BBC Hulton Picture Library; *Figures 2.5 and 2.6* Mansell; *Figure 5.1* The Warden and Fellows of New College, Oxford; *Figure 5.2* L.F. Hirst, *British Encyclopaedia of Medical Practice*, Butterworth; *Figure 5.3* P. Ziegler, *The Black Death*, Collins, 1970; *Figure 5.6* courtesy of Royal Statistical Society; *Figure 5.7* from *The Plague Reconsidered*, Local Population Studies, 1977; *Figure 5.8* Known and probable foci and areas of plague 1959–1979, in *Weekly Epidemiological Record*, vol. 55, no. 32. World Health Organisation, 1980; *Figure 6.2* USSR Academy of Science; *Figures 6.5 and 6.6* J. Hatcher, *Plague, Population and The Economy*, Macmillan, London and Basingstoke, 1977; *Figures 7.1, 7.3, 9.1, 9.2 and 9.3 (a)* courtesy of The Royal Society of Medicine; *Figures 7.4 and 7.5* E. Vayda, A decade of surgery in Canada, England and Wales and The United States, in *Archives of Surgery*, vol. 117, © 1982 American Medical Association; *Figure 8.1* E. Mandel *et al.*, Excessive surgery in hysteria, in *Journal of the American Medical Association*, vol. 151, © 1953 American Medical Association; *Figures 9.3 (c) and (d)* courtesy of Wellcome Institute.

Answers to self-assessment questions

Chapter 2

1 The quotations illustrate that, in order to develop knowledge that was of some practical use, one had to engage in close observation of the real world and detailed experimentation. Armchair speculation and purely abstract theorising led nowhere.

2 (a) This is an example of the classical monistic form of medical theory in which diseases are merely the surface manifestation of one underlying condition. It is that single condition which needs treatment and there is a single remedy for it — here, the Gamboge Pill. Since the pill is purgative, Morrison is using a form of humoral theory as opposed to the alternative form of medical monism which saw tensions in the solid part of the body as the cause of all illness.

(b) (i) Sydenham's method of disease classification was based on direct observation of patients and close attention to their signs and symptoms. The technique was a big advance but only worked well for those limited number of diseases with a distinctive cluster of outward signs. The accurate classification of other diseases had to wait until clinical findings were systematically compared with data from post-mortems; a method developed in the eighteenth century by Morgagni and others.

(ii) In medieval medicine, the focus was on the sick individual. There was thought to be one disease-state, and illness was a complete disturbance of the individual's bodily balance. Each illness episode affected different individuals in distinctive ways. The medieval doctor, therefore, went to the patient's bedside to learn about their individual characteristics. By contrast, Sydenham's work represents the beginning of the modern belief that there are many different types of disease, each of which has characteristic effects. Sydenham, therefore, went to the bedside to study the general properties of particular diseases, not the particular qualities of particular individuals.

(c) Bernard's theory stresses the vital importance of maintaining the equilibrium of various body systems.

However, although classical medical theory also concerned itself with theories of internal balance, it differed in two vital respects. First, it emphasized the importance of the individual, the sickman — everyone had their own individual balance. Modern medical science minimises the differences between individuals. Second, Bernard's theory of homeostasis rested on a detailed knowledge of anatomy, physiology and localised pathology. This new theory of internal equilibrium was based on detailed knowledge of the part played by individual components such as organs, glands and cells in maintaining that balance.

3 Therapeutic nihilism was a nineteenth-century medical doctrine which held that most supposed cures were useless and some possibly harmful. The best remedy was, therefore, to let nature take its course, a line of action which appealed strongly to those who believed that most disease was self-limiting.

4 Doctors relied, where they could, on an appeal to the academic authority of the classical tradition; on advertising and publishing their own books; on personal authority; on a good bedside manner; on claims to be scientific; on social status and wealth. Of these, a mere doctor's wealth is unlikely to have made much impact on a prince. However, since the major development of medical science from the late nineteenth century onwards, medical authority has come to rest increasingly on the appeal to science. Thus, whereas many doctors once laid particular stress on their personal authority and skill, their contemporary authority, even in private practice, depends more on an appeal to a collective body of scientific knowledge.

5 (a) Both focus on the role of the individual medical hero, and the book title emphasises extraordinary scientific triumph ('breakthrough') and heroic struggle ('saga'). All three elements are central components of the Whig theory.

(b) The idea that scientific knowledge could be cumulative, that each generation could build upon the discoveries of the past, was radically new. Previous eras had looked back to the past in reverence. After the Renaissance, people began to look instead to the future and the discoveries and opportunities that it might bring.

Chapter 3

1 The message refers to the theory that contemporary life is bad for you and that health resides in a return to a 'natural' state.

2 (a) Official entry into the sick role was made much harder. (b) It suggests that the extent to which people may enter the sick role varies according to social and economic circumstances.

3 Several different traditions were mentioned in the text: (i) descendants of eighteenth-century monistic systems, such as homeopathy; (ii) classical traditions from other cultures, e.g. acupuncture; (iii) folk traditions, e.g. herbalism; (iv) magico-religious traditions, e.g. faith-healing.

4 (a) Mad. (b) The cause is seen as supernatural; the treatment involves direct mediation with supernatural beings; and the healer also is both in the natural and supernatural realms. (c) Casting out evil spirits still occurs, both in African societies and in the West — exorcism.

5 The product claims to 'impart a vigour to the whole system'. Humoral theory saw disease as a disturbance of the whole system.

6 Both types of therapeutic nihilism involve the beliefs that medical intervention may do more harm than good and that most medical therapy is ineffective. However, Illich concedes that some progress has been made. On the other hand, he also introduces an entirely new criticism — that these successes, relatively trivial though he thinks they are, have led to modern society becoming addicted to medicine and in danger of being controlled by it.

Chapter 4

1 Measles and smallpox had been around sufficiently long in the Old World for a process of mutual accommodation to occur between the Spanish population and the microorganisms that cause these diseases. By contrast, the Indians and the microorganisms had never previously met. It took several generations before an equivalent accommodation could be reached in the New World.

Chapter 5

1 The chronicler was writing fifty years later, probably making use of anecdotal evidence and anxious to write a good story. The deaths of the abbot and 6 monks on one

precise date (and a date consistent with our other knowledge of the spread of the disease) may well be correct, and derived from a record made at the actual time. The numbers 34 and 50 may be less reliable. It does, however, seem possible that the death-rate in close-knit communities might be higher than the average mortality of 30 per cent.

2 (a) *Yersinia pestis* seems to have established a degree of accommodation with some species of wild rodents, which act as a kind of natural reservoir, a 'homeland' for the bacillus. There is regular disease here, but rarely of the devastating kind that affects some of its other hosts who have a far more unstable relationship with the bacillus. The rat serves as an intermediate host between the wild rodents and the human species. Although a rodent, it does not live in the wild but close to human habitation. It can, therefore, serve as a means by which a third host, the flea, can pass from the infected wild rodents to human beings. The flea, which lives on blood, feeds off all three other hosts and in doing so circulates the bacillus among them. Finally, the human's role in this chain of transmission is as crucial as any. Although human beings have not developed any major degree of accommodation with the bacillus and cannot therefore act as stable home and source of food, the human capacity to develop extensive, rapid and global forms of travel has meant that the bacillus has been able to establish new bases in colonies of burrowing rodents all over the world. Humans have unwittingly transmitted the disease to rodents just as rodents have unwittingly transmitted it to them.
   (b) Endemic disease.
   (c) Plague did not become established in the human population because, at the very start of the third pandemic, the human species identified the bacillus that was the immediate cause of the infection and began to develop counter-measures. The key steps here were the identification of the bacillus; the discovery of the role of rats, fleas and wild rodents; the creation of public health measures against infected rats; the development of vaccines; and the eventual discovery of antibiotics, which proved a cure for those who had contracted the disease.

3 Quarantine measures are effective against the pneumonic form of the plague, but have less impact on the bubonic and septicaemic forms, since these are transmitted by fleas and rats.

4 That the epidemic was so marked in the Scandinavian countries, despite their relatively cool climates, suggests that pneumonic plague may have been responsible for much of the mortality there. The lower mortality in central Europe might possibly be due to the fact that it is in direct contact with the Asian plague foci. Some degree of immunity might already have developed in the rodent and

human populations. (The other possibility is that bubonic plague, with its lower mortality rate, may have a greater capacity for transmission across great distances by land than the more virulent pneumonic form.)

Chapter 6

1 The scale and speed of the third pandemic reveal the importance of endogenous factors (factors internal to the human social world). For example, plague had never before reached the Americas and could only do so via the new steamships. On the other hand, McNeill's argument that the pandemics were due solely to endogenous factors such as improved communication and trade seems implausible. By 1894 major international networks of communication had existed for a long time. Why should plague break out precisely then and move as fast as it did? An exogenous factor, such as mutation in the bacillus, seems more plausible. To summarise, both biological and social factors need to be examined.

2 There is reference to four theories. Boccaccio refers directly to beliefs that the plague was sent by God or was the product of astrological influence. His description of the public health measures refers implicitly to two further theories. The removal of 'filth' was based on miasmatic theories and the introduction of quarantine measures derived from contagonist beliefs.

3 There is good evidence that infectious diseases such as plague can have highly destructive effects on a society. Not only may the survivors become demoralised and terrified, but some may engage in savage acts of violence — such as the persecution of the Jews in the fourteenth century. In the longer run, it may threaten or destroy an entire society. But there may also be beneficial effects, though these are much debated. The population of England fell dramatically during the first century of the second pandemic and wage levels rose accordingly. This may possibly have stimulated a variety of technical and economic innovations. And, whatever the uncertainties, it seems most unlikely that those who died were 'the best'. Plague seems to have struck at people quite indiscriminately.

Chapter 7

1 (a) The mid-nineteenth century; (b) the twentieth century.

2 The following critical points can be made: (i) Are women actually choosing this operation or are they instead being forced into it? (ii) Is it that richer women can afford it, or is it that private surgeons are particularly interested in their riches? (iii) What evidence is there that hysterectomy is a serious investment against cancer? (iv) Might there perhaps be other more harmful consequences of this operation?

3 The statement assumes that we know what is and what is not a 'necessary' operation. But this is precisely what is disputed. For some people, hysterectomy is almost never justified; for others, there is a very obvious need for it. Since there is no agreement on this subject, it is impossible to make accurate calculations of the number and cost of unnecessary operations — at least in the case of hysterectomy.

4 (a) Government policy in allocating resources; clinicians' judgement; women's judgement. (b) Clinicians' judgement; Government policy; women's judgement. (c) Several other possible factors were mentioned in the chapter: surgeon's training; gender relationships; the method of payment; national income level; the degree of surgical monopoly in the United Kingdom; the number of surgeons.

Chapter 8

1 Hysteria, by definition, mimics organic illness. The only evidence for it is, therefore, purely negative: the diagnosis of hysteria is arrived at by the absence of any sign of physical disease. There are no positive indications for the condition. Moreover, it is always possible that the doctor might be wrong, might have missed some underlying organic illness.

2 A feminist critic might argue that the real explanation lay not so much in the doctor's medical training as in the general male prejudice against women which informed that training. They might also argue that it is not surprising if some women respond histrionically to male domination.

3 A conflict theory of hysteria would argue that because most women in most societies are in a subordinate position, they are obliged to adopt an overtly submissive manner, however much they dislike this. It is, therefore, no surprise that some women's self-image is 'inauthentic'. Moreover, since on the conflict theory, hysteria can be both a refuge and a revenge, we might expect such women to exhibit 'a kind of ruthless wilfulness' and to be hard for psychotherapists to deal with.

Chapter 9

1 Men could use Genesis in several ways. First, women could be told that it was their religious duty to obey their husbands. Second, men could argue that it was a man's duty not to listen to his wife. Third, men could point out that it was a woman who was responsible for the suffering in this world — 'cherchez la femme'. Women could be portrayed as temptresses leading innocent men into sin.

2 (a) This is a mixture of biological and mental theories. There are references to organic explanations (the emphasis on firm or soft bodies) and to quasi-mental explanations

(the invisible 'animal spirits' which 'can be seen only with the eyes of the mind').

(b) A degree of blame is hinted at in the last sentence. Women are portrayed as idling about while men do the hard work. There is also a suggestion that women go in for imaginary suffering because they do not know what real suffering is like.

3 (a) It was written in 1970. (b) Galen and Harvey (both men) assume that regular intercourse with a man is essential for a woman's physical and mental health. Galen thought it was medically important that women be 'receptive and eager to the advances of their husbands'. Likewise, Harvey spoke of the virtue which proceeds from the male *in coitu* (during sex). Novak's textbook does not suggest that women's health depends on this. However, sex is again portrayed as something which men do to women, and for which the latter should be grateful. And if they are not, they should see their doctor immediately. In other words, now as 2500 years ago, some male doctors try to regulate women's sexuality in ways that serve male interests.

Entries and page numbers in **bold type** refer to key words which are printed in *italics* in the text.

Index